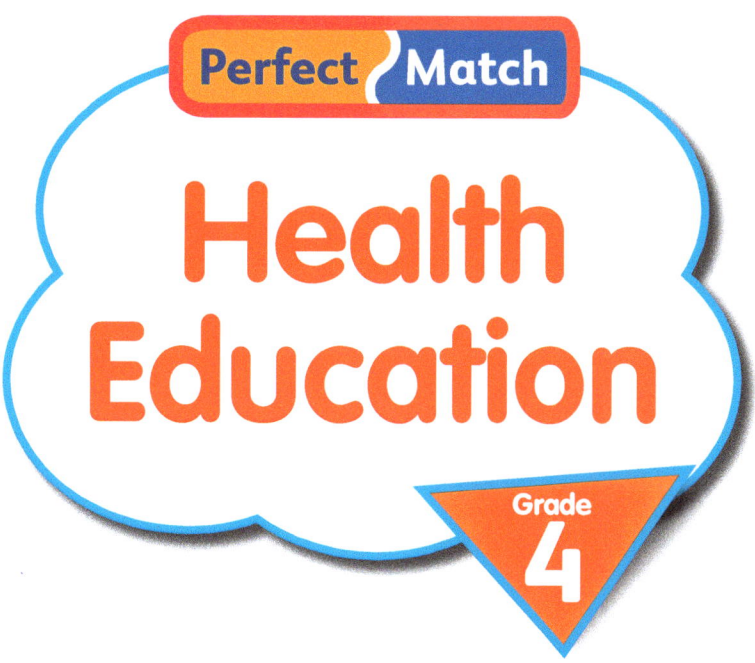

Dr Michael Chia

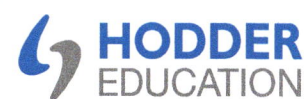

The Publishers would like to thank the following for permission to reproduce copyright material.

Photo credits
sai0112©123RF.COM; Andrey Bourdioukov©123RF.COM;scanrail©123RF.COM; Aleksey Boldin©123RF.COM; Iakov Filimonov©123RF.COM

Hachette UK's policy is to use papers that are natural, renewable and recyclable products and made from wood grown in well-managed forests and other controlled sources. The logging and manufacturing processes are expected to conform to the environmental regulations of the country of origin.

ISBN: 978 981 47 6775 0

© Dr Michael Chia 2018

This edition published in 2018 by
Hachette Singapore Private Limited
Published from 2023 by Hodder Education,
An Hachette UK Company
Carmelite House
50 Victoria Embankment
London EC4Y 0DZ
www.hoddereducation.com

Impression number   10 9 8 7 6 5
Year   2023

All rights reserved. Apart from any use permitted under UK copyright law, no part of this publication may be reproduced or transmitted in any form or by any means, electronic or mechanical, including photocopying and recording, or held within any information storage and retrieval system, without permission in writing from the publisher or under licence from the Copyright Licensing Agency Limited. Further details of such licences (for reprographic reproduction) may be obtained from the Copyright Licensing Agency Limited, www.cla.co.uk

Printed and bound by CPI Group (UK) Ltd, Croydon, CR0 4YY

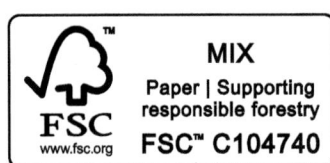

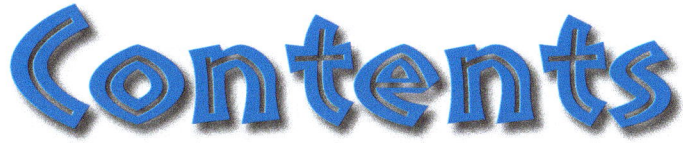
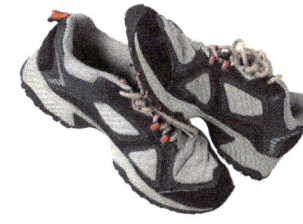

Physical Health

Lesson	Title	Page
1	Keeping Fit With Regular Exercise	3
2	Developing A Healthy Heart	5
3	Building My Bones	7
4	Eating My Way To Good Health	9
5	Making Healthy Choices	11
6	Hand And Foot Hygiene	13
7 & 8	Too Smart To Start	17
9	My Precious Sight	21
10	Myopia Or Short-Sightedness	23
11 & 12	Do Away With Tooth Decay	25

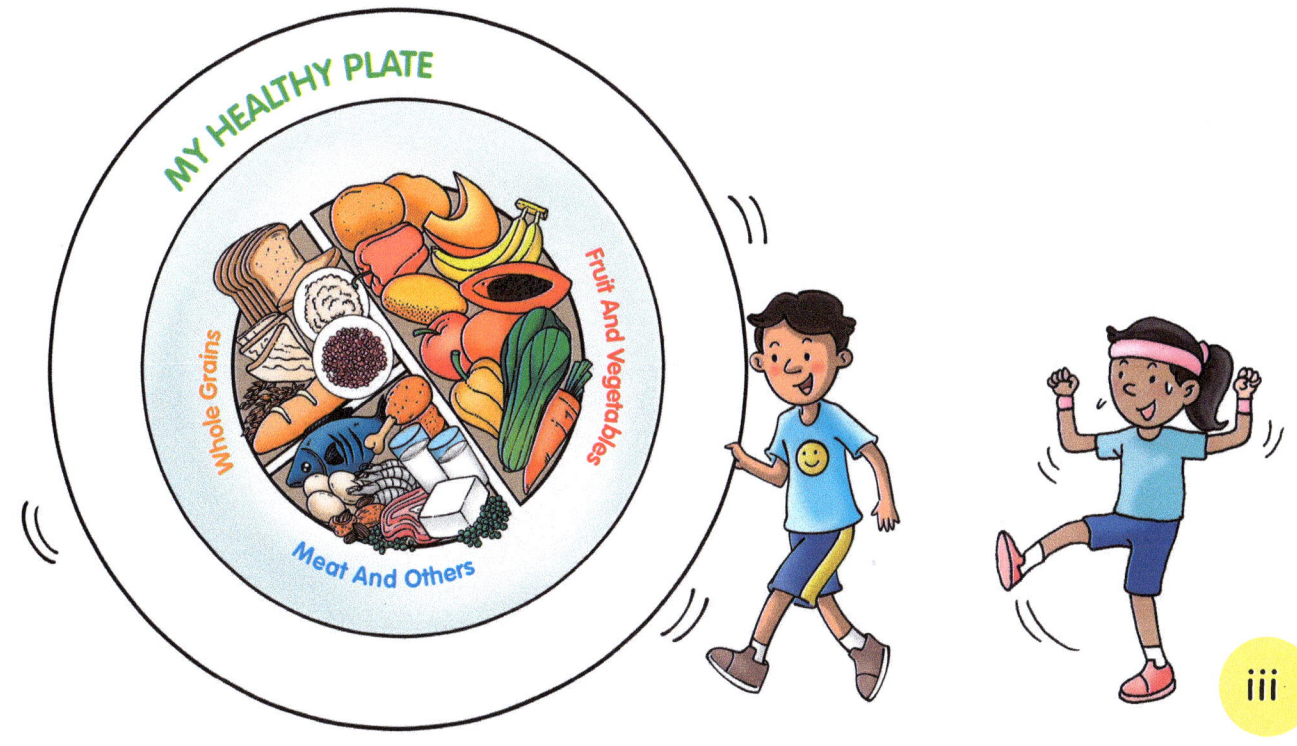

Environment And Your Health

Lesson	Title	Page
1	Being Wise About Water	31
2	Dangerous Water	33
3	Safety At The Pool	35
4	Fire Hazards In The Home	37
5	Is Your Home Fire-Safe?	39
6	Fire Strikes	41
7	What's In Your Food?	43
8	Practise Good Food Hygiene	45
9	Let's Practise Food Safety	47

Emotional And Psychological Health

Lesson	Title	Page
1	Building My Confidence	51
2	Our Strengths and Weaknesses	53
3	Try Something New	55
4	Caution, Danger Ahead!	57
5	Protect Yourself	59
6	Beware Of Offers From Strangers	61
7	What Should I Do?	63

Learning Log	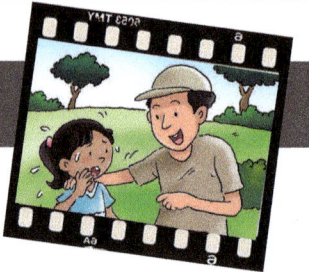	65-70

Introduction to the Pupil's Book

The **Perfect Match** Primary Health Education Pupil's Book is a full-colour textbook-cum-activity book. It contains lessons based on topics from the three dimensions in Health Education: Physical Health, Environment and Your Health, and Emotional and Psychological Health.

The book is organised by dimension and is presented in the order stated above. The pages in each dimension are colour-coded for easy reference.

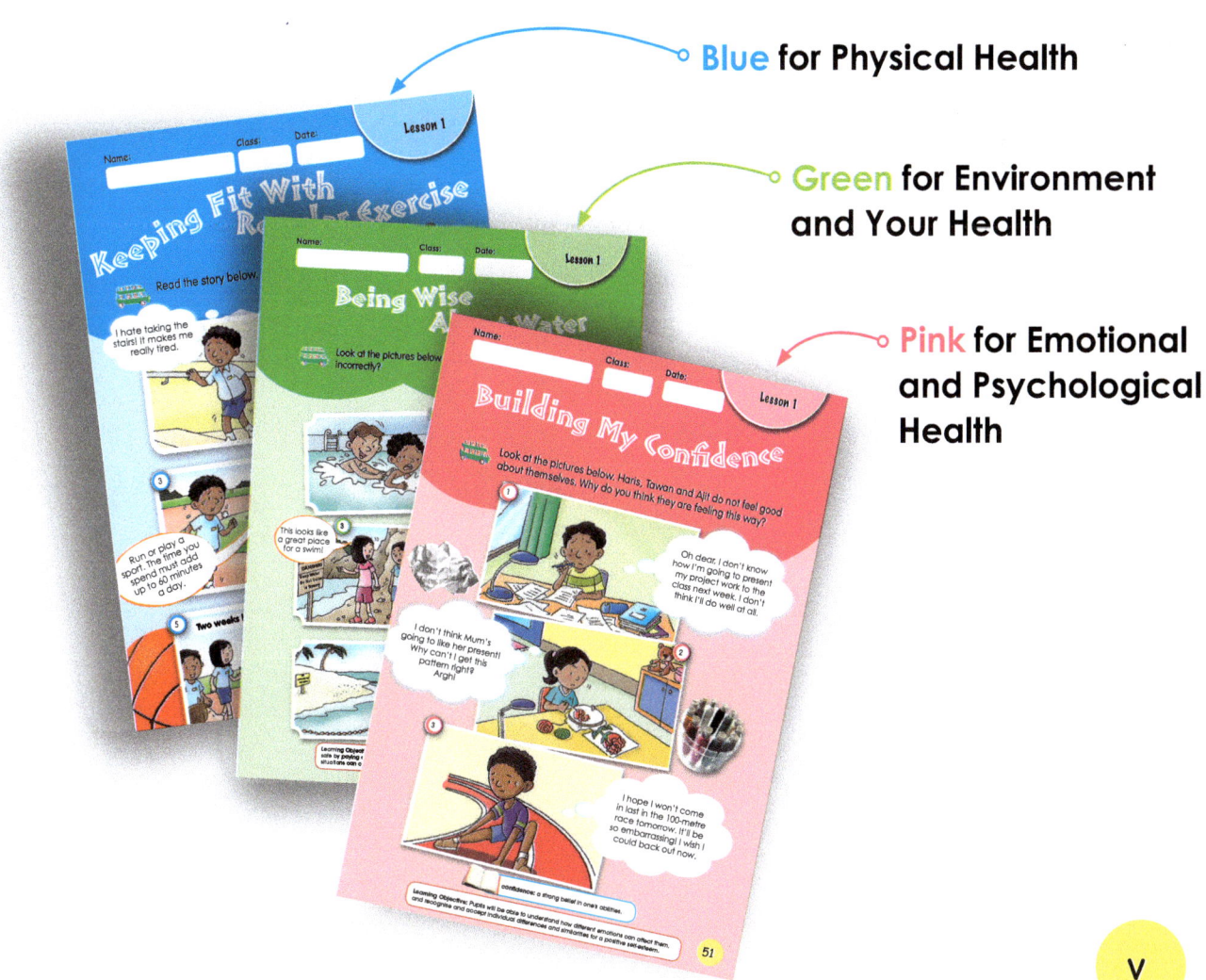

Blue for Physical Health

Green for Environment and Your Health

Pink for Emotional and Psychological Health

The Pupil's Book contains a variety of activities such as role plays, surveys, songs, matching exercises and craft work. In addition, there is a mix of activities requiring work in pairs, in groups or with the class.

Four icons indicate the nature of the activity to be conducted.

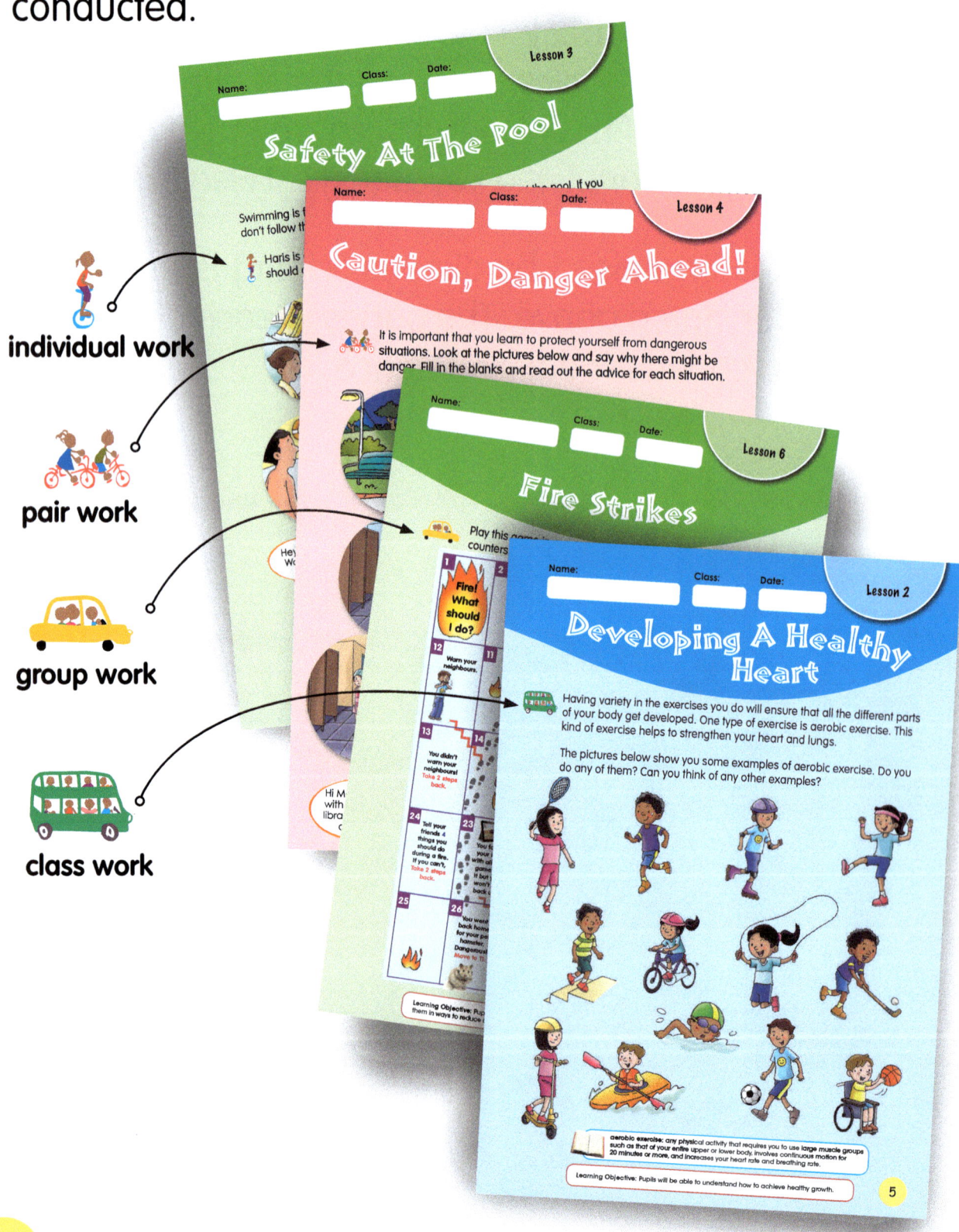

Difficult terms mentioned in the text are explained through a feature signaled by the dictionary icon.

The learning objective(s) for each lesson is/are listed for parents and teachers and found at the opening page of each lesson.

A dictionary icon signals the explanation of any difficult term(s) found on the page.

The learning objective(s) for each lesson is/are indicated at the opening page of each lesson.

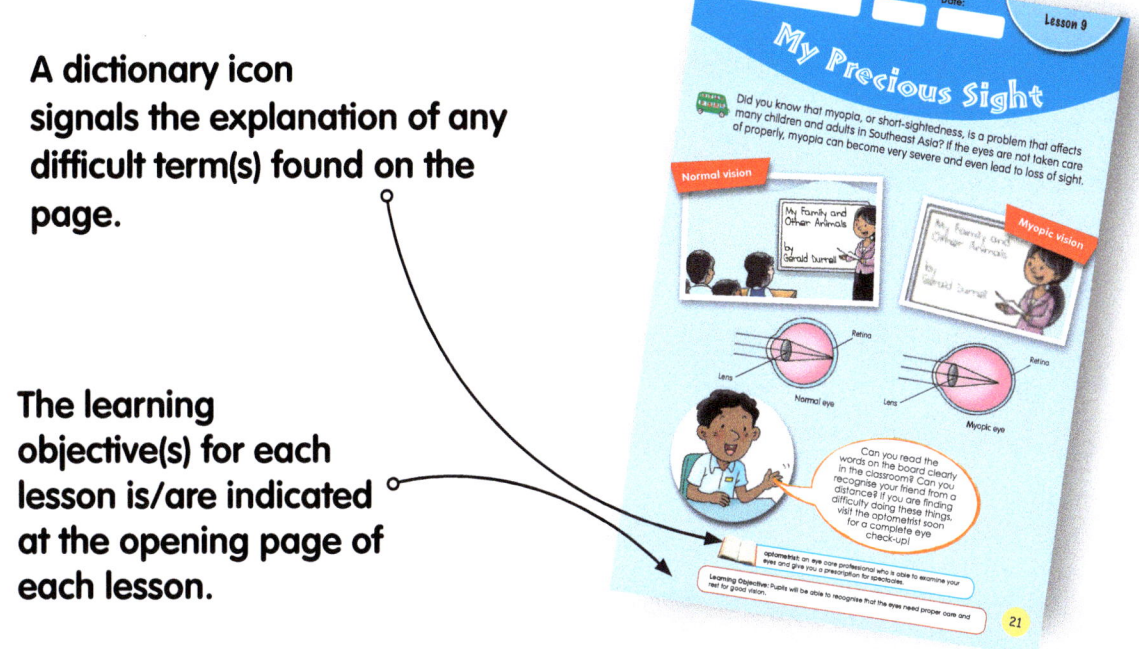

Pupils may be given additional notes or worksheets reproduced from the Teacher's Resource in their book.

A Note on Short Forms: In the first three books, short-forms of verbs are avoided as early users of the language may not have knowledge of them. In Books 4, 5 and 6, these contractions are present throughout so that the language flows more naturally and pupils can become more acquainted with real English use.

A Learning Log has been added at the end of the book to give opportunity for reflective learning.

vii

Meet the Superfriends!

The materials in the Perfect Match Primary Health Education Pupil's Book revolve around six superfriends from some of the ASEAN countries. These six friends will accompany the pupils in the learning process as they move from Book 1 to 6. The first letters of their names – Haris, Eileen, Ajit, Lam, Tawan and Harold – form the word 'h-e-a-l-t-h'.

Taking the cue from the World Health Organization (WHO) to build 'a better and healthier future for people all over the world', the superfriends come together from different ASEAN countries to help young people like themselves develop healthy habits to ensure a better future.

This health series aims to help pupils start early in health education, to keep themselves well physically, psychologically and emotionally. In addition, they will also learn to behave responsibly in order to enhance the environment in their home countries.

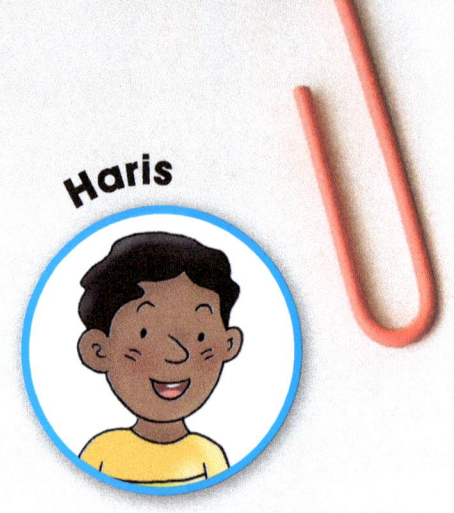

Haris

Appearance:
A well-built Malaysian boy.

Interest:
Being with people.

Special quality:
He's the wise one.

Motto:
Happiness is caring for others and making them happy!

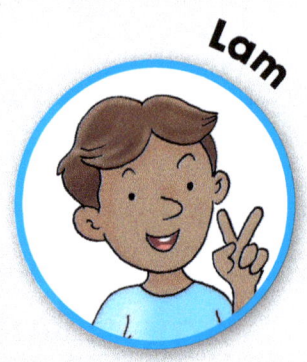

Lam

Appearance:
A tall and lean Vietnamese boy.

Interests:
Learning and new ideas.

Special quality:
Good-natured and patient.

Motto:
Always give and share what you have

Eileen

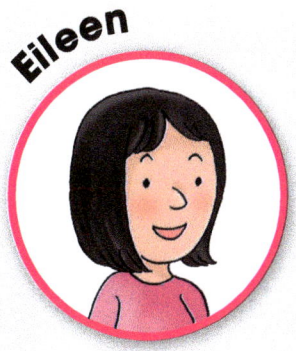

Appearance:
A tall slim Singaporean girl.

Interest:
Loves Maths and Science and knows a lot about computers.

Special quality:
She's the brainy one.

Motto:
IT makes the world go round!

Ajit

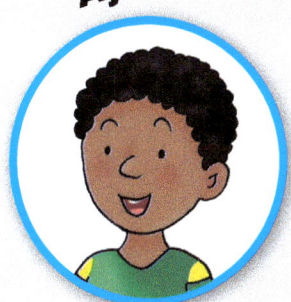

Appearance:
A good-looking Malaysian boy.

Interests:
Reading and learning languages.

Special quality:
He's the articulate one.

Motto:
Observe and listen to understand better!

Tawan

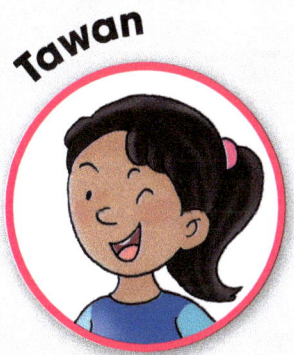

Appearance:
An athletic and sporty Thai girl.

Interests:
Art and sports.

Special quality:
Strong in character, fun-loving and witty.

Motto:
Love and live life!

Harold

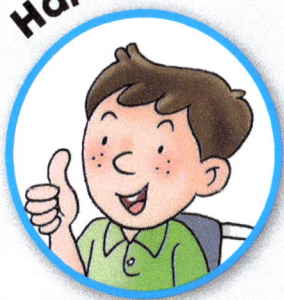

Appearance:
A smiley Singaporean boy.

Interest:
Music.

Special quality:
Confident, determined and focused.

Motto:
Reach for the impossible!

About The Author

Dr. Michael Chia is Professor of Paediatric Exercise Science at the Physical Education & Sports Science Group in the National Institute of Education (NIE), Nanyang Technological University (NTU). He is an established author in the field of Health Education, Physical Education and Sport Science. His health education publications include *Healthy Well* and *Wise: Take PRIDE For A Life of Wellness, Invest in Better Health* and *Treks: All Aboard!*.

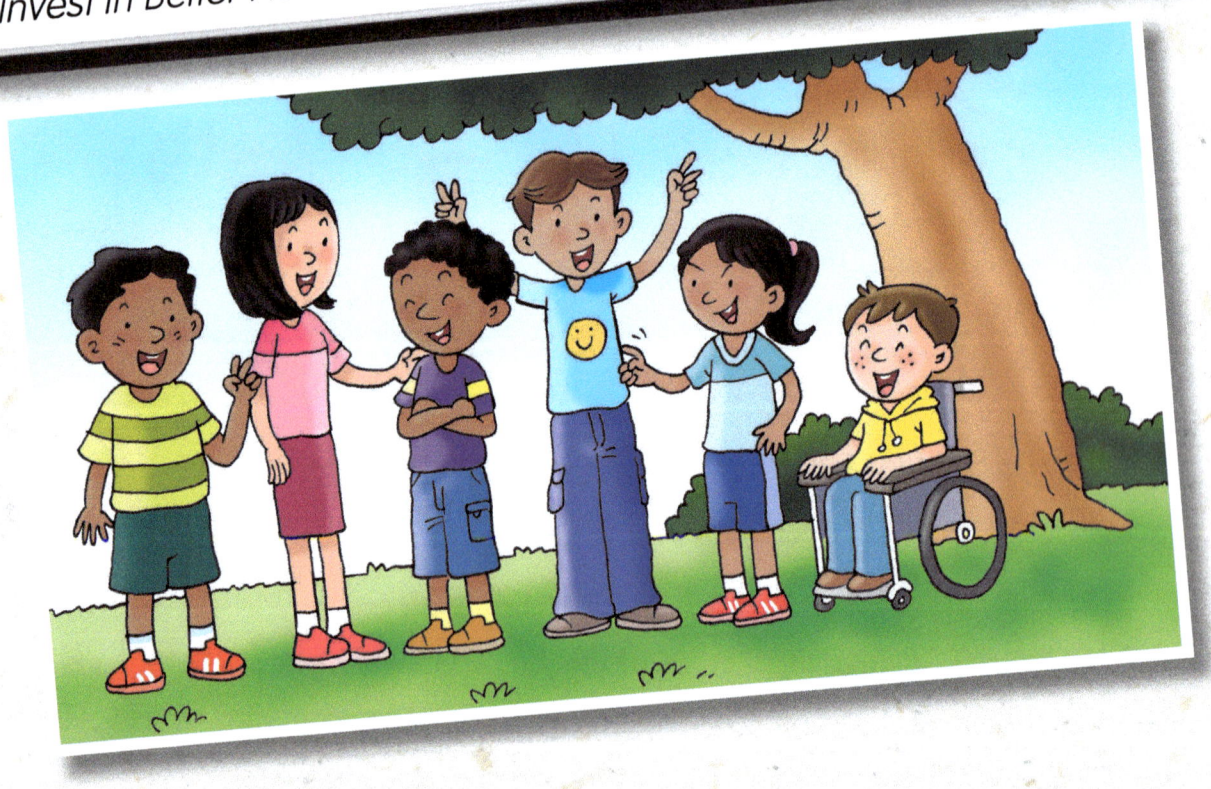

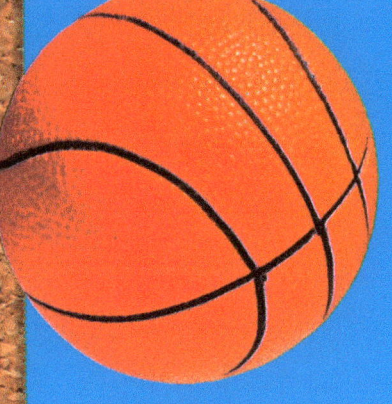

Physical Health

In this section, you will learn:

- why exercise is important;
- more about My Healthy Plate;
- the importance of personal hygiene;
- about harmful substances;
- how to take care of your eyes; and
- about tooth decay and ways to prevent it.

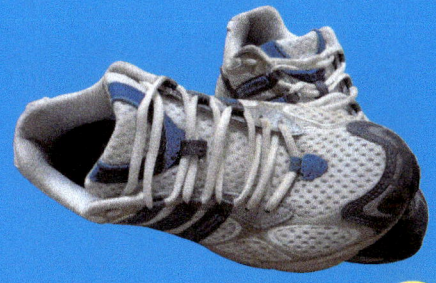

Name: Class: Date:

Lesson 1

Keeping Fit With Regular Exercise

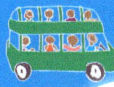 Read the story below.

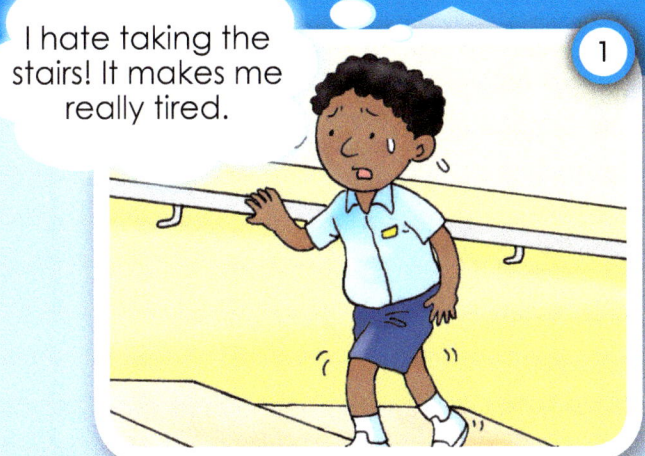

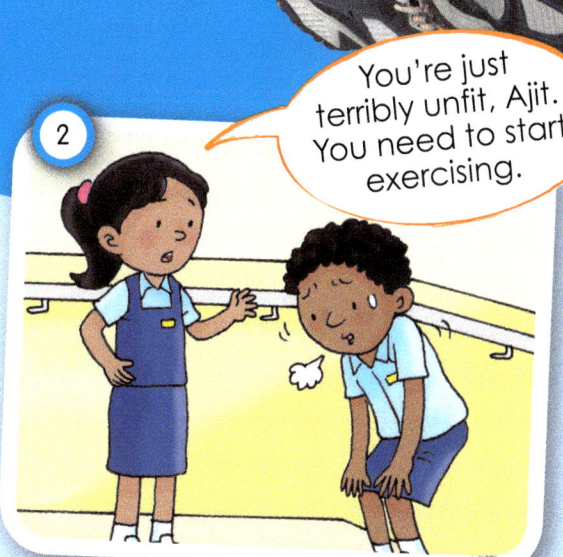

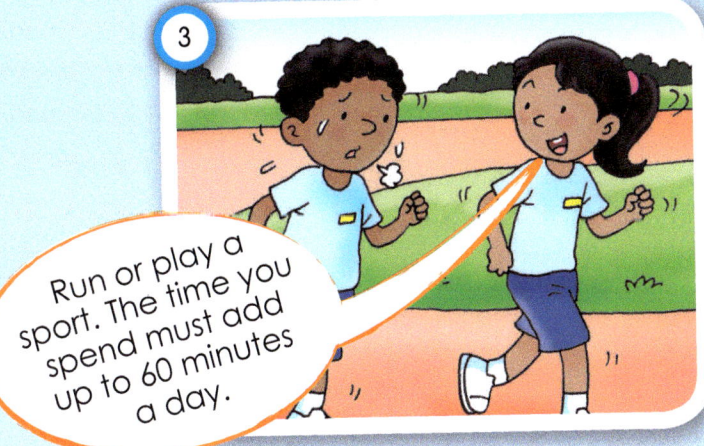

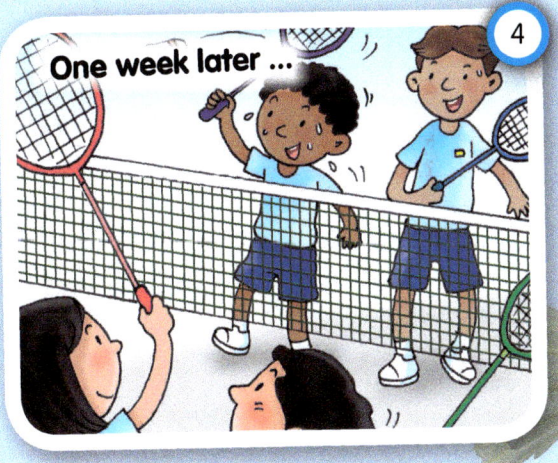

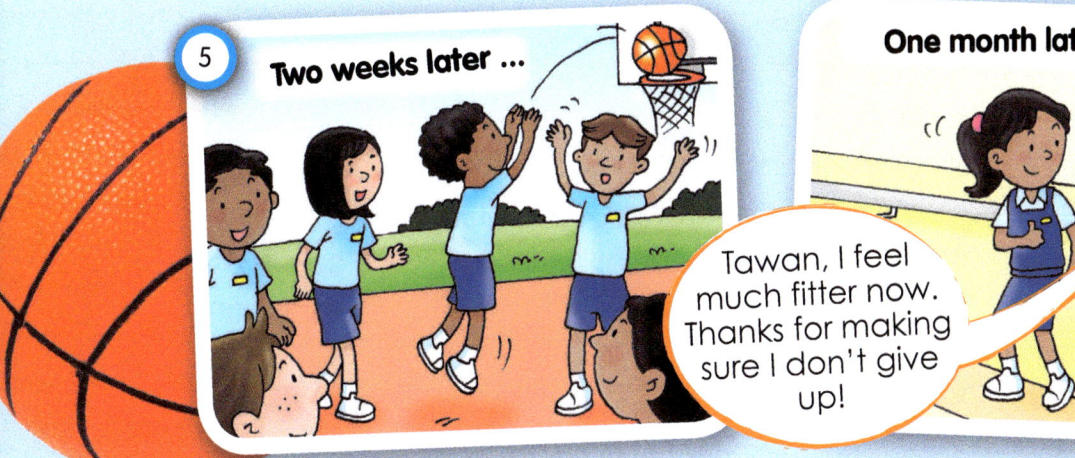

Learning Objective: Pupils will be able to understand how to achieve healthy growth.

3

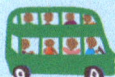 Take a look at the exercise schedule that Tawan helped Ajit to plan for his first week of exercise. What do you notice?

Day	Activities				Total Time
MON	Walking to school 7 – 7.15am	P.E. 8 – 8.30am	–	–	45min
TUE	Walking to school 7 – 7.15am	Playing catching Recess (20min)	Walking home 1.30 – 1.45pm	–	50min
WED	–	–	Basketball CCA 2 – 3pm	–	1h
THU	Walking to school 7 – 7.15am	Badminton Recess (15 min)	Walking home 1.30 – 1.40pm	Cycling 4 – 4.20pm	1h
FRI	–	P.E. 8 – 9am	Soccer 2 – 2.15pm	–	1h 15min
SAT	Swimming 9 – 10am	–	Frisbee 4 – 4.30pm	–	1h 30min
SUN	–	–	Rollerblading 3 – 4.35pm	–	1h 35min

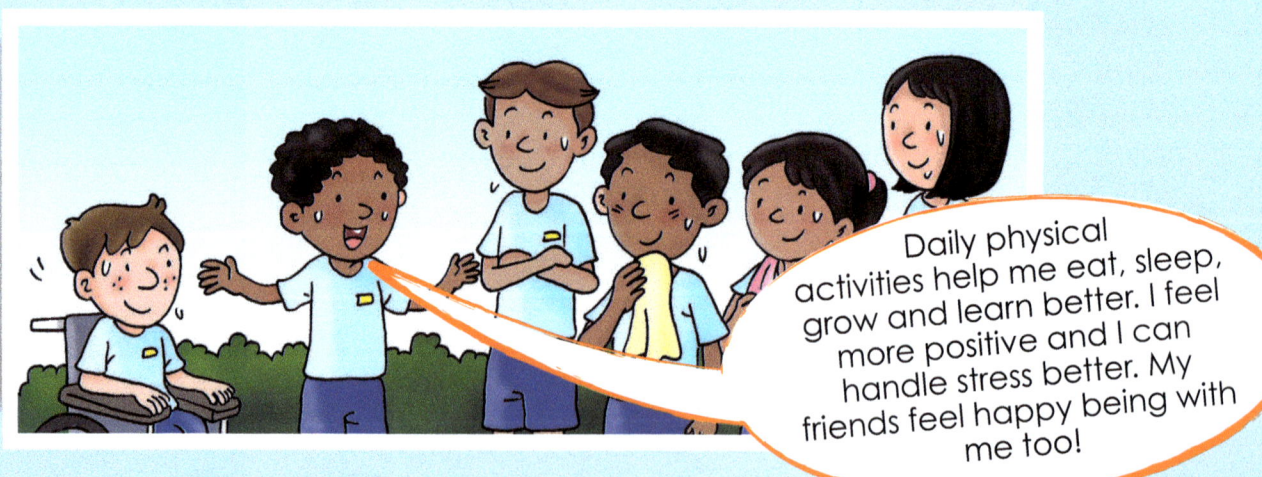

Daily physical activities help me eat, sleep, grow and learn better. I feel more positive and I can handle stress better. My friends feel happy being with me too!

Regular exercise makes you fit by strengthening your bones, muscles, heart and lungs. When you are fit, you will have more energy to do the things that you enjoy. You can also do a moderate-to-vigorous physical activity (MVPA) such as vigorous dancing, sprinting or fast swimming. Try to have some MVPA at least 3 times a week.

regular exercise: for children, this means at least 60 minutes of MVPA or vigorous exercise every day. It does not need to be in a single stretch.

moderate-to-vigorous physical activity (MVPA): an activity that causes the heart to beat faster, and breathing to deepen and quicken. When you are engaged in MVPA, you will have enough breath to talk but not enough for you to sing.

Name: Class: Date:

Lesson 2

Developing A Healthy Heart

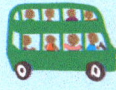 Having variety in the exercises you do will ensure that all the different parts of your body get developed. One type of exercise is aerobic exercise. This kind of exercise helps to strengthen your heart and lungs.

The pictures below show you some examples of aerobic exercise. Do you do any of them? Can you think of any other examples?

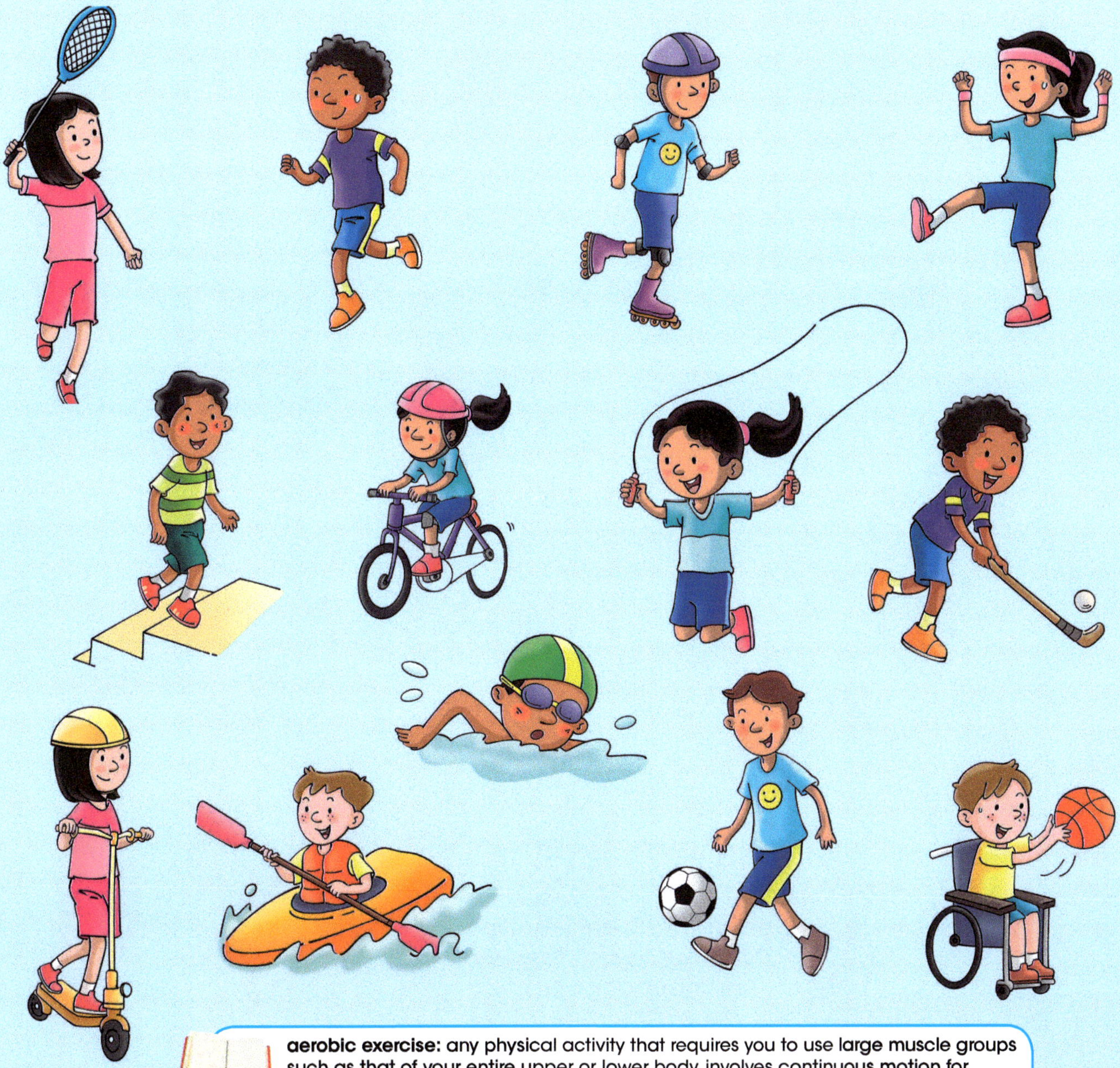

aerobic exercise: any physical activity that requires you to use large muscle groups such as that of your entire upper or lower body, involves continuous motion for 20 minutes or more, and increases your heart rate and breathing rate.

Learning Objective: Pupils will be able to understand how to achieve healthy growth.

5

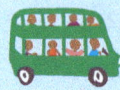

Aerobic exercise makes your heart pump faster and harder. Since the heart is a muscle, all this exertion makes it stronger. The stronger your heart is, the fitter you are!

The Pulse Rate Chart is a guide that tells you how hard you should make your heart work when you exercise. While you are exercising, use this chart to check that your pulse rate falls within the green zone.

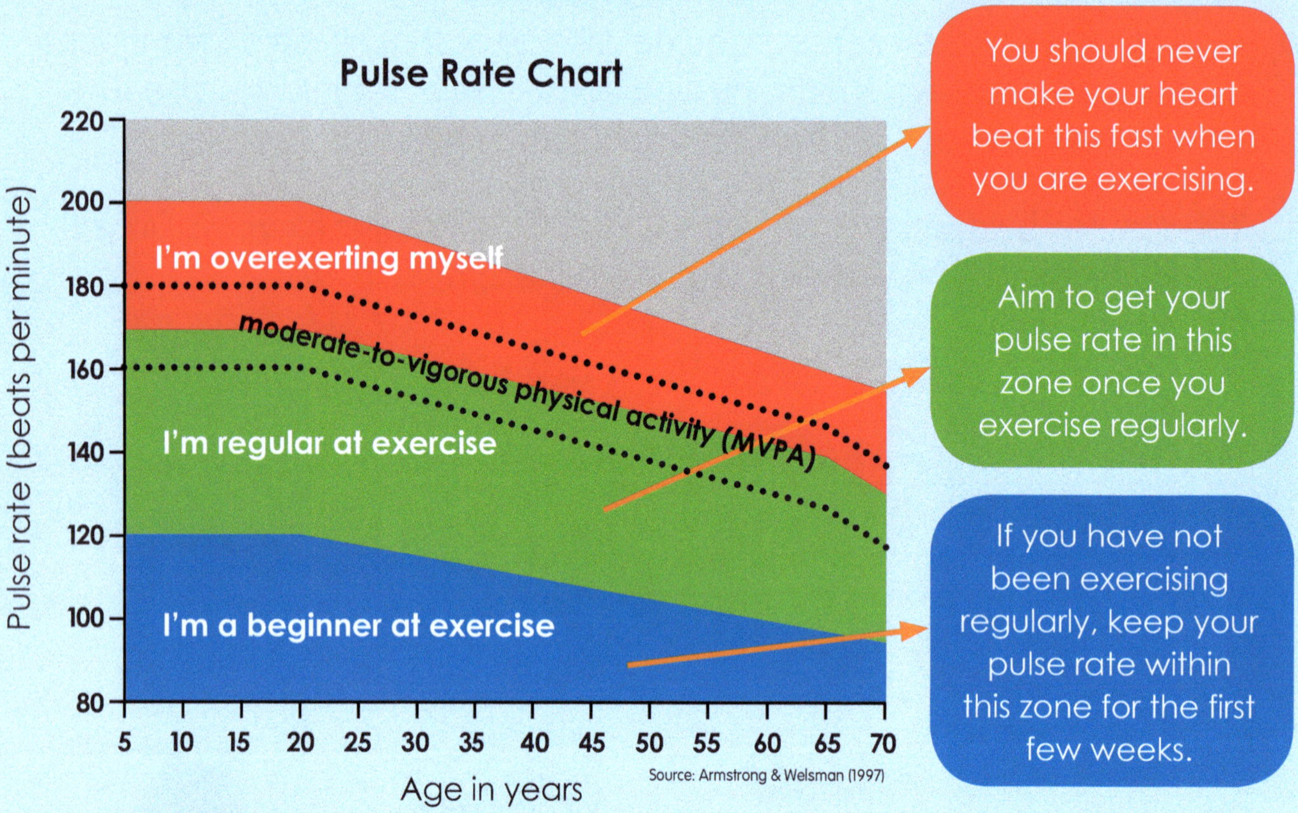

Pulse Rate Chart

- I'm overexerting myself
- moderate-to-vigorous physical activity (MVPA)
- I'm regular at exercise
- I'm a beginner at exercise

Source: Armstrong & Welsman (1997)

You should never make your heart beat this fast when you are exercising.

Aim to get your pulse rate in this zone once you exercise regularly.

If you have not been exercising regularly, keep your pulse rate within this zone for the first few weeks.

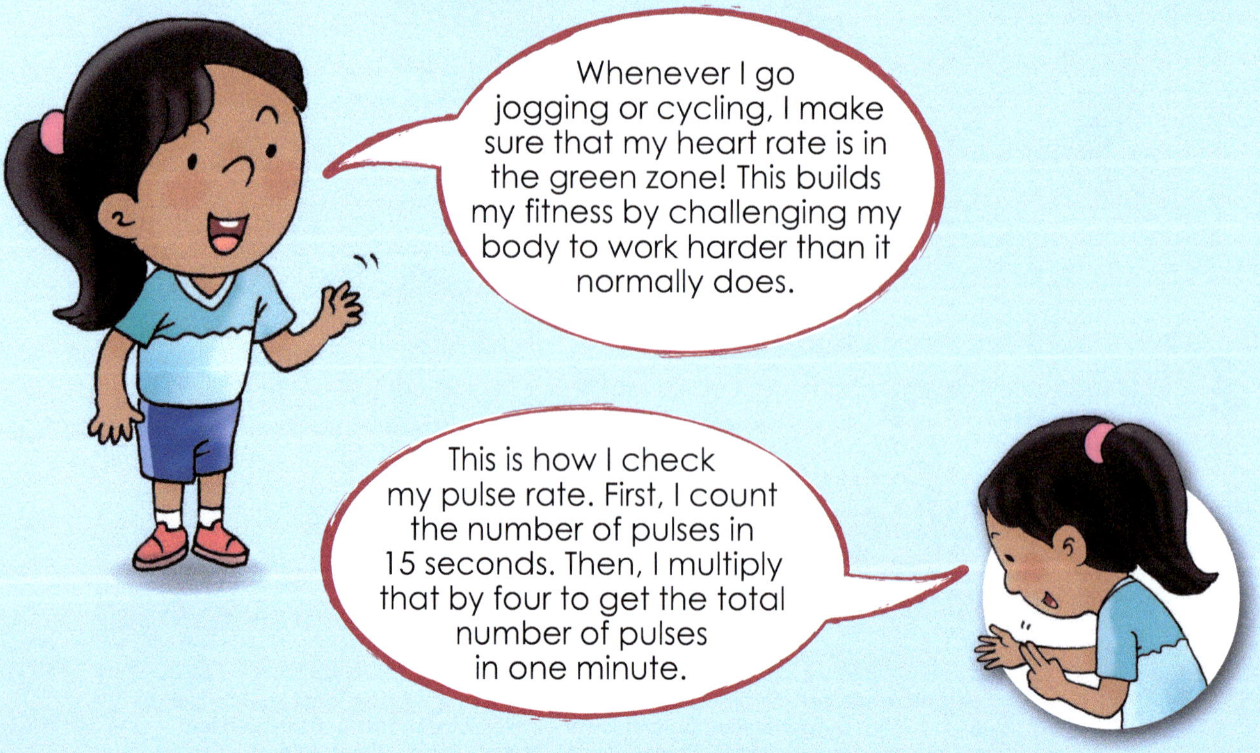

Whenever I go jogging or cycling, I make sure that my heart rate is in the green zone! This builds my fitness by challenging my body to work harder than it normally does.

This is how I check my pulse rate. First, I count the number of pulses in 15 seconds. Then, I multiply that by four to get the total number of pulses in one minute.

pulse rate: the number of times your heart beats in one minute.

Name: **Class:** **Date:** Lesson 3

Building My Bones

In the different exercises that you do, be sure to include weight-bearing exercise. This type of exercise builds and strengthens your bones and muscles.

You now know about the two main types of exercise that will help you grow strong and healthy. Listen to your teacher read what Harold, Haris and Tawan have to say about their favourite activities. Place a tick (✓) under the part of their bodies in which they are building fitness. In the last column, decide if each activity is 'weight-bearing', 'aerobic', both or neither.

Activity	Heart and lungs	Bones	Muscles	Type of exercise
Push-ups				
Running				
Cycling				

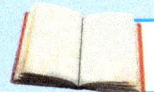

weight-bearing exercise: any physical activity that involves your bones and muscles working against gravity to carry your entire body weight on your feet and legs.

Learning Objective: Pupils will be able to understand that good eating habits and exercise are necessary to develop and maintain healthy growth.

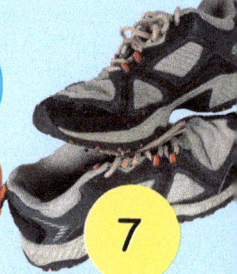

7

Like muscles, your bones become stronger when they have to support your body weight. The pressure that is applied on them increases their density. Bones are strong when they have high density. This means that they will not break easily even if you have a bad fall.

Tawan's grandmother is in the hospital because she fell down and broke her hip. She has osteoporosis. This means that her bones break easily because they have very low density.

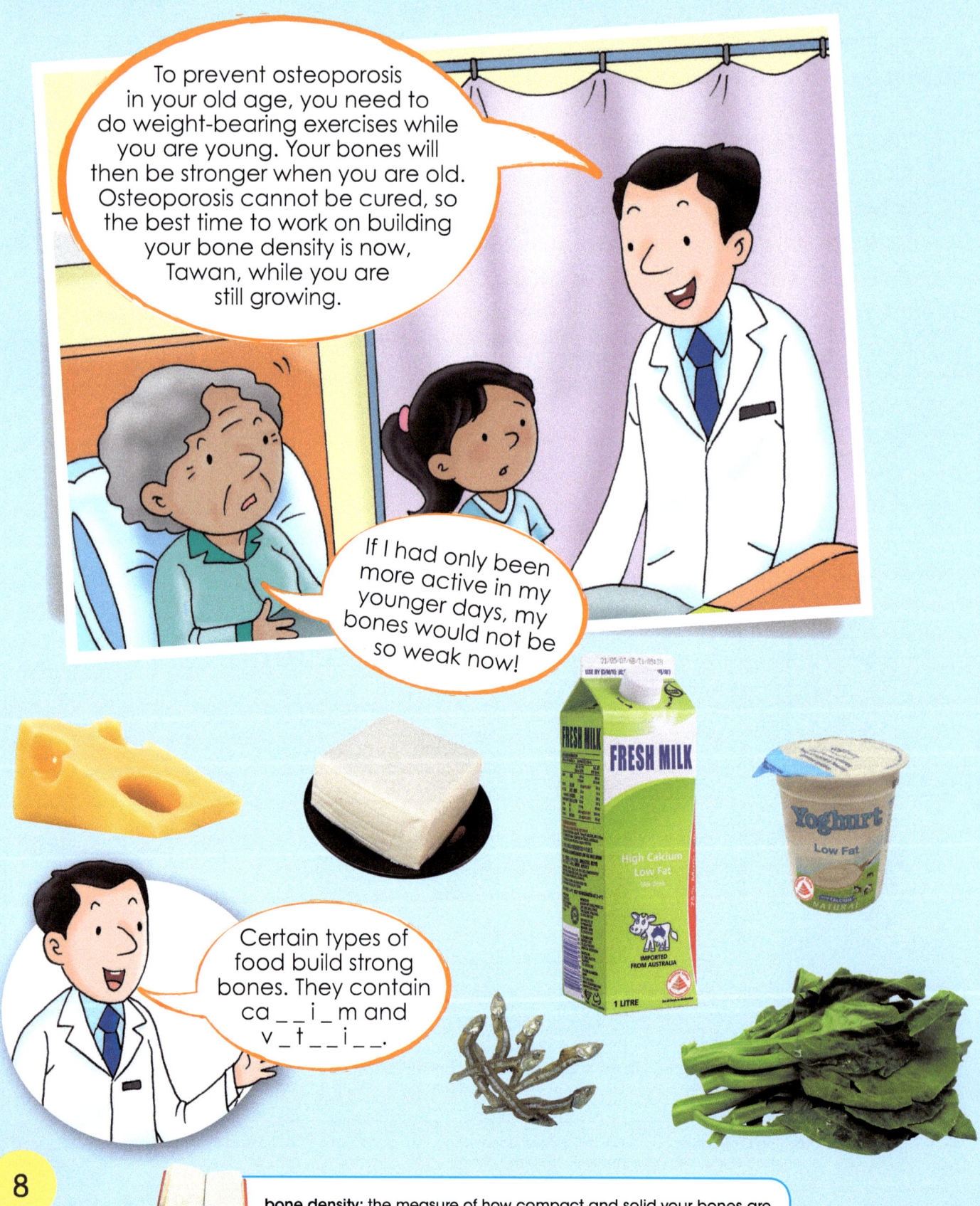

To prevent osteoporosis in your old age, you need to do weight-bearing exercises while you are young. Your bones will then be stronger when you are old. Osteoporosis cannot be cured, so the best time to work on building your bone density is now, Tawan, while you are still growing.

If I had only been more active in my younger days, my bones would not be so weak now!

Certain types of food build strong bones. They contain ca _ _ i _ m and v _ t _ _ i _ _.

bone density: the measure of how compact and solid your bones are.

Name: Class: Date:

Lesson 4

Eating My Way To Good Health

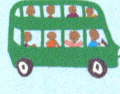 To eat healthily for each meal, My Healthy Plate recommends that we have half a plate of fruit and vegetables, a quarter-plate of meat or others, and a quarter-plate of whole grains.

My Healthy Plate here shows examples of one serving for each food type. It also tells you the number of servings you need each day.

WHOLE GRAINS
Energy-giving food
How much to consume **each day**?
- 5 to 6 servings (5 servings for children who are less active.)

Examples of one serving:
- ½ bowl of rice
- 2 slices of bread
- ½ bowl of noodles or spaghetti
- 1 thosai
- 1 ½ cups of cereal

Eat ONE serving daily of brown rice or wholemeal bread as part of the 5 to 6 servings.

FRUIT
Protective food
How much to consume **each day**?
- 2 servings

Examples of one serving:
- 1 medium banana
- 1 wedge of pineapple, papaya or watermelon
- 1 glass of pure fruit juice (no sugar added)
- 10 grapes or longans

VEGETABLES
Protective food
How much to consume **each day**?
- 2 servings

Examples of one serving:
- ¾ mug cooked leafy vegetables
- ¾ mug cooked non-leafy vegetables
- ¼ round plate cooked mixed vegetables

MEAT AND OTHERS
Protective food
How much to consume **each day**?
- 2 servings

Examples of one serving:
- 1 palm-sized (child's hand) portion of meat, fish or chicken
- 5 medium prawns
- 3 eggs
- 2 cheese slices

In addition to the 2 servings, drink 250 to 500ml of milk each day.

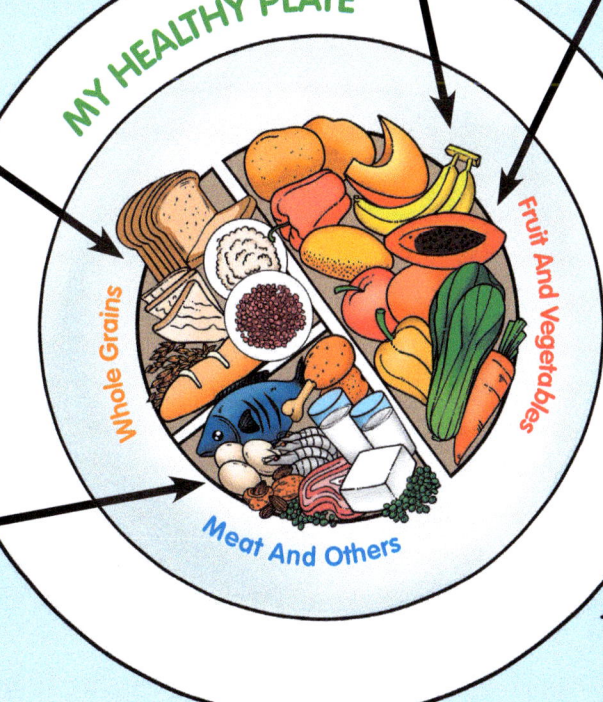

serving: one portion of food.

Learning Objective: Pupils will be able to understand how to make healthy food choices to obtain and maintain healthy growth.

 Try your hand at planning a day's meals for your partner. Refer to the requirements on My Healthy Plate on the previous page.

Write your food items in the plan for the three plates: breakfast, lunch and dinner. Make sure the servings for the three meals add up to the daily servings requirements:
- Fruit and vegetables: 2 + 2 servings
- Whole grains: 5 to 6 servings
- Meat and others: 2 + 1 (milk) servings

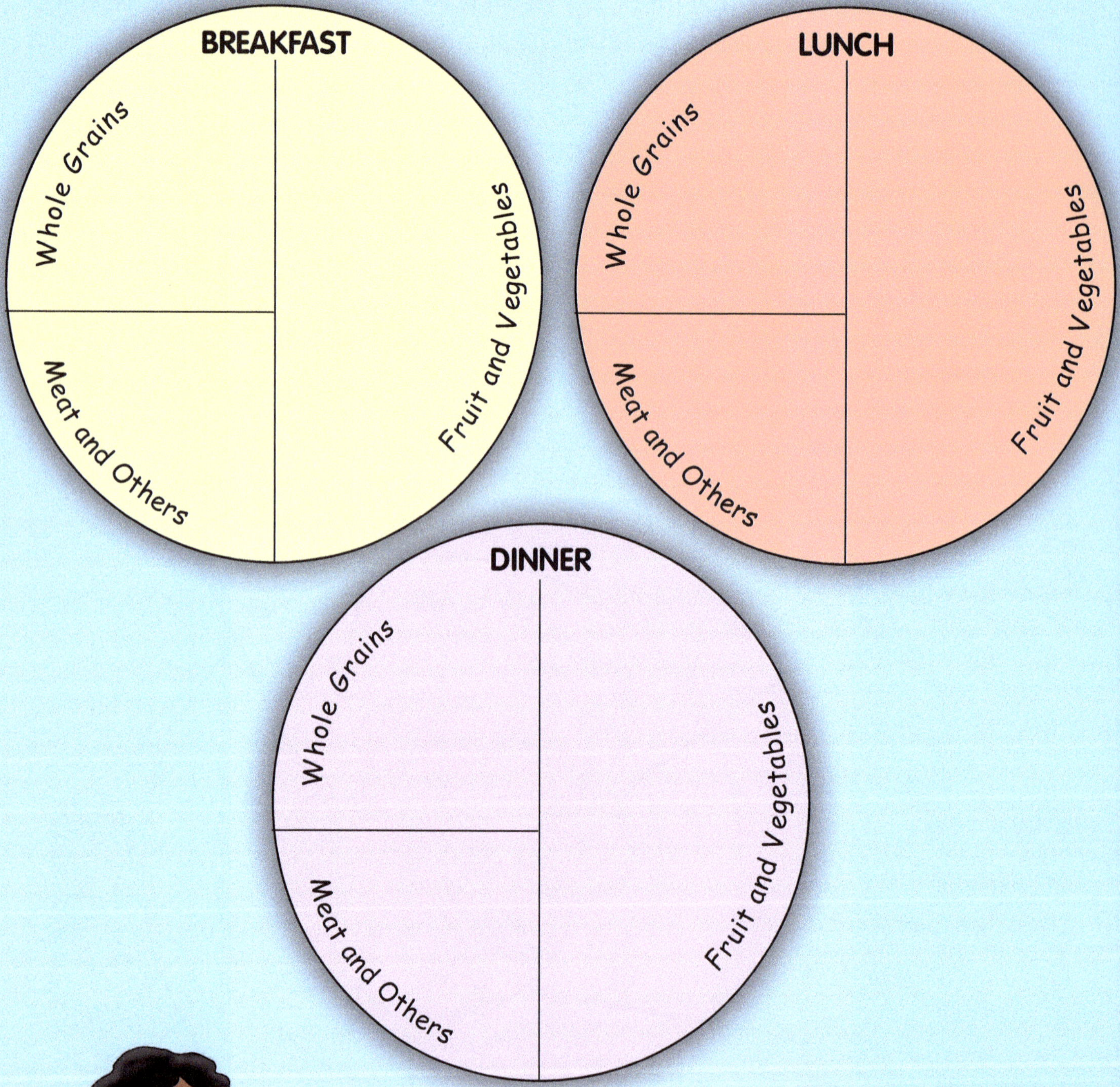

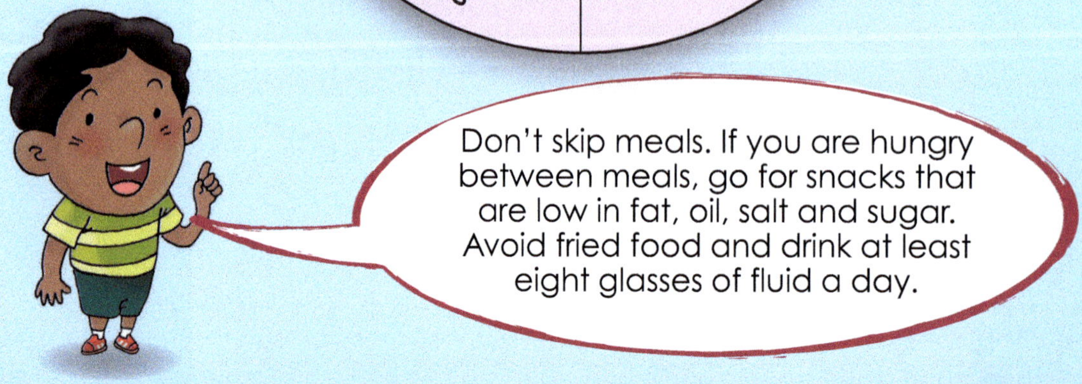

BREAKFAST

LUNCH

DINNER

Don't skip meals. If you are hungry between meals, go for snacks that are low in fat, oil, salt and sugar. Avoid fried food and drink at least eight glasses of fluid a day.

10

Name: Class: Date: **Lesson 5**

Making Healthy Choices

Choose food that is high in fibre. Fibre can be found in fruit and vegetables as well as food items like wholemeal bread. On the other hand, fat, oil and sugar should be taken in small amounts although they help make food tasty. The superfriends want to help you make the right choices. Read what they have to say about the effects of these two different groups of food.

> Choose food that is high in fibre and be sure to drink at least eight glasses of fluid a day. This will give you healthy bowel movement that cleanses your body of waste products and toxins.

> If you eat a lot of food that contains high amounts of fat, oil, salt and sugar, you could end up with health problems such as high cholesterol and high blood pressure. These could lead to heart disease and stroke!

cholesterol: a waxy, fat-like substance found in cells in the human body. There is good and bad cholesterol. Bad cholesterol sticks to the walls of blood vessels and makes it difficult for blood to flow through.

Learning Objective: Pupils will be able to understand how to make healthy food choices to obtain and maintain healthy growth.

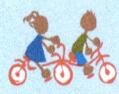 Are you making the right choices in the way you eat and in the food you eat? Take the quiz below to find out how much you know. Circle 'T' if you think the statement true and 'F' if you think it is false.

1. You do not need to have breakfast as long as you have a hearty lunch. T / F

2. Wholemeal bread is good for you. T / F

3. You should eat calcium-rich food because it helps build strong bones and teeth. T / F

4. There is no problem eating only one meal a day. You only have to eat enough to meet your daily nutritional needs in that one meal. T / F

5. A balanced diet keeps you healthy. T / F

6. It is all right to have fried chicken every day, as long as you only have two or three servings of it each day. T / F

7. Fresh fruit and vegetables are healthy snacks. T / F

8. You should drink more than eight glasses of water a day. T / F

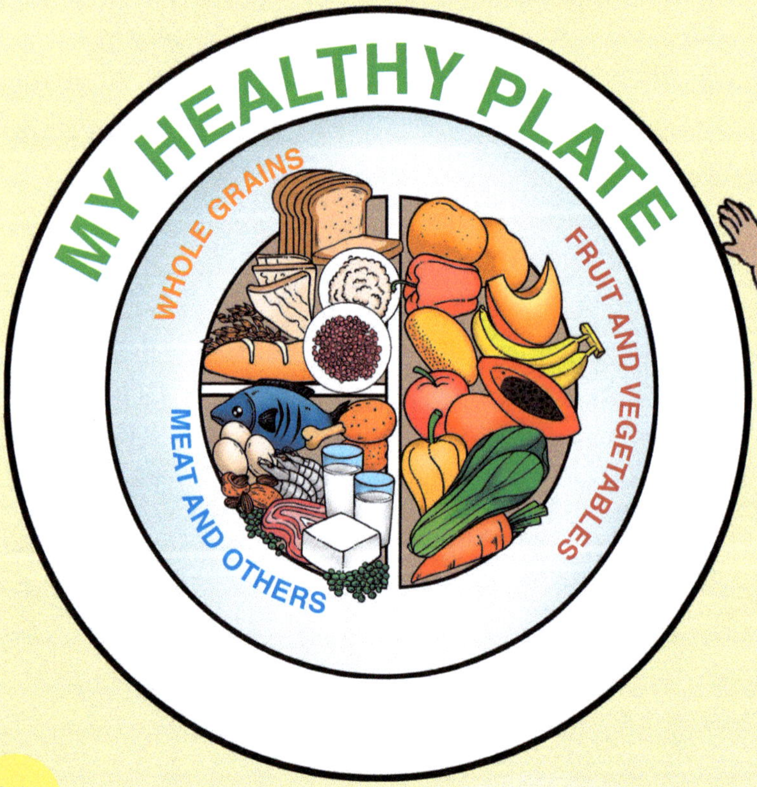

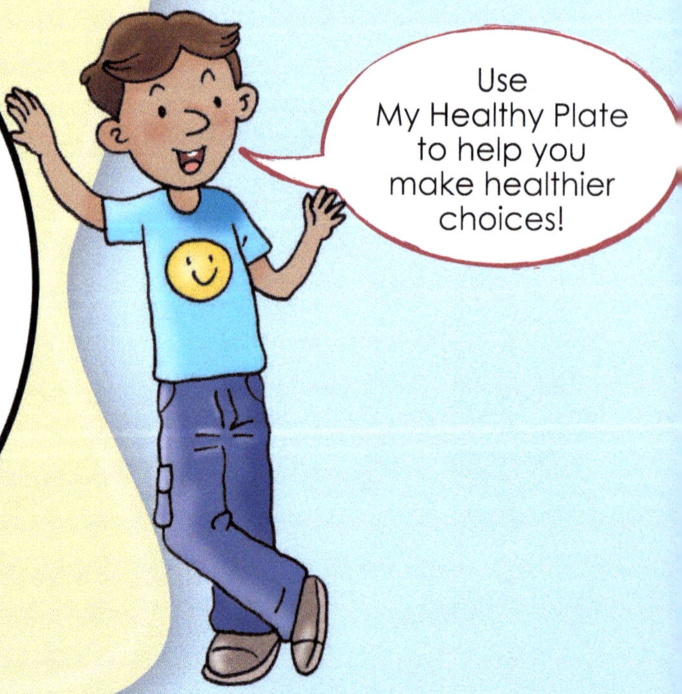

Use My Healthy Plate to help you make healthier choices!

Hand And Foot Hygiene

Lesson 6

Name: ____ Class: ____ Date: ____

All that you touch and hold can put germs on your hands. When you touch food or rub your eyes, germs can be transferred and you can fall sick. It is therefore important to wash your hands regularly.

 Are you and your friends practising good hand hygiene? Interview your partner to find out! Place a tick (✓) in the box if the statement is true for him or her.

How Clean Do You Keep Your Hands?

My partner's name is _____ .

He/she always washes his/her hands…

1. before eating. ☐
2. after playing with pets. ☐
3. after playing outdoors. ☐
4. after using the toilet. ☐
5. before handling food. ☐
6. after clearing the wastepaper basket. ☐
7. after playing with toys. ☐
8. after handling sports equipment. ☐
9. after wiping his/her nose, mouth or feet. ☐
10. after touching lift buttons, door knobs, railings, etc. ☐

Learning Objective: Pupils will be able to understand how to establish daily habits for caring for their bodies in order to maintain or improve health and prevent illnesses.

Another way to keep your hands and feet clean and neat is to trim your nails regularly. This will prevent them from collecting dirt and germs from all the objects that you touch and places that you visit!

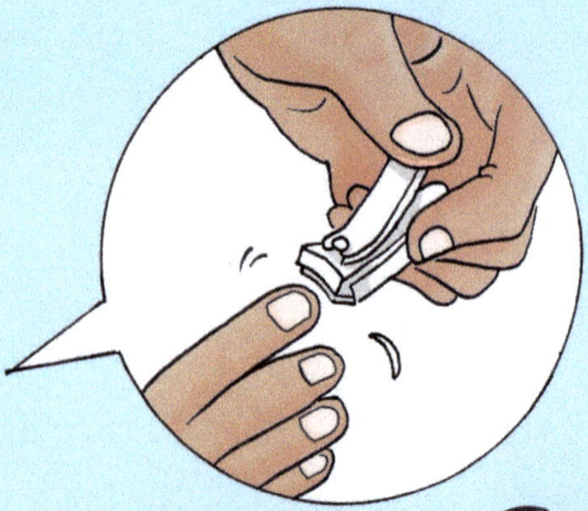

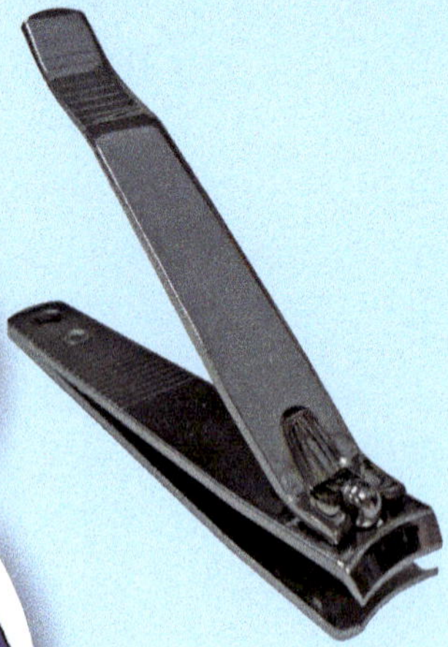

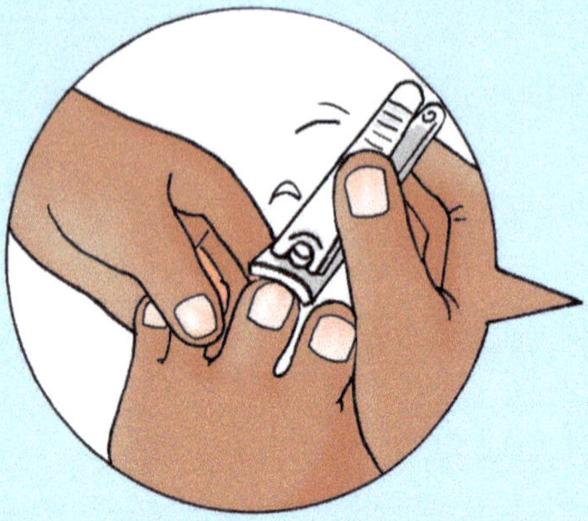

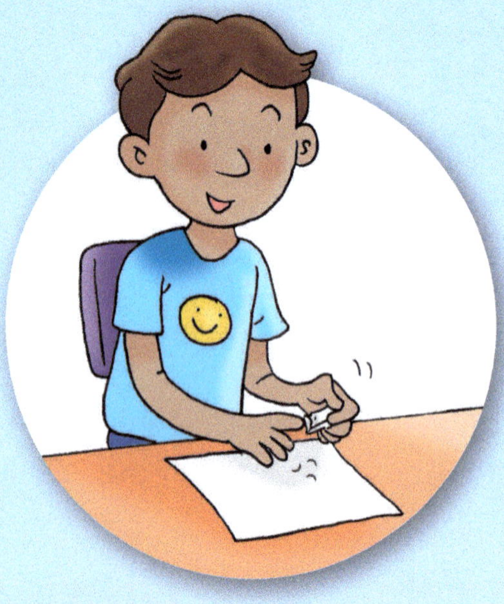

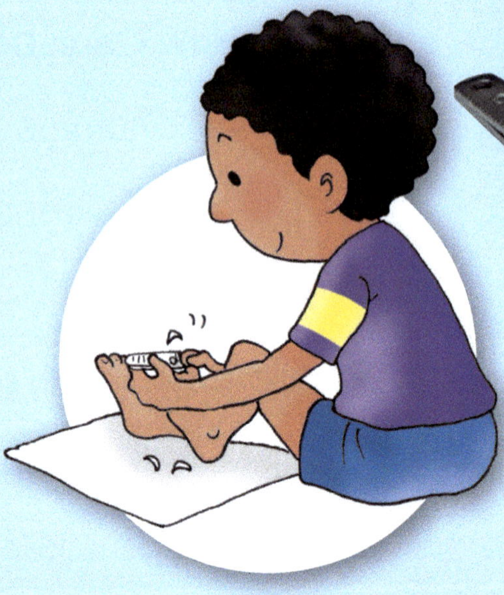

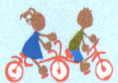 Besides trimming your toenails and washing your feet, how else can you keep your feet clean and odour-free? Unscramble the letters to find out!

Change your _ _ _ _ _ every day
(ksosc)
and wash your _ _ _ _ _ _ _ _ _ _ _ _
(ochlso hesos)
every weekend!

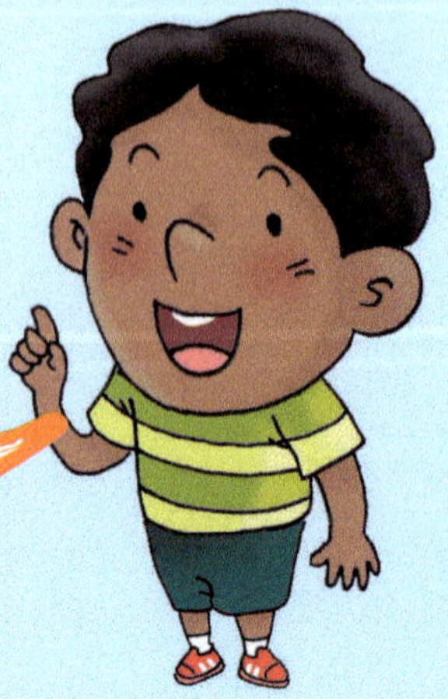

Here's how you should wash your hands and feet.

Hand-washing

Seven Steps To Hand Hygiene

1.
2.
3.
4.
5.
6.
7.

1. Get into a group of four. Go through the handwashing procedure. Memorise the seven steps. (This should be done without water and soap.)
2. Choose one person to be the prompter. The prompter can look at the book to check if the group is following the seven-step procedure correctly.
3. The other three will take turns to lead the group.
4. Each leader will demonstrate one step at a time. If the leader gets the step right, the rest will follow. If the leader gets it wrong, no one should follow. The prompter can whisper to the leader what the correct thing to do is.
5. There will be three rounds of 'hand-washing'.

Foot Hygiene

 Fill in the blanks to complete the instructions for pictures 1 to 6.

1. _ _ sh your feet daily with s _ _ p and wa _ _ r.

2. D _ y your feet well, especially between the to _ _.

3. Ch _ _ g _ your socks d _ _ ly.

4. Keep your shoes dry. Loosen the laces and a _ r them when not in use.

5. Avoid walking ba _ _ f _ _ ted outdoors.

6. Wash your s _ _ _ _ _ shoes every we _ _ en _ .

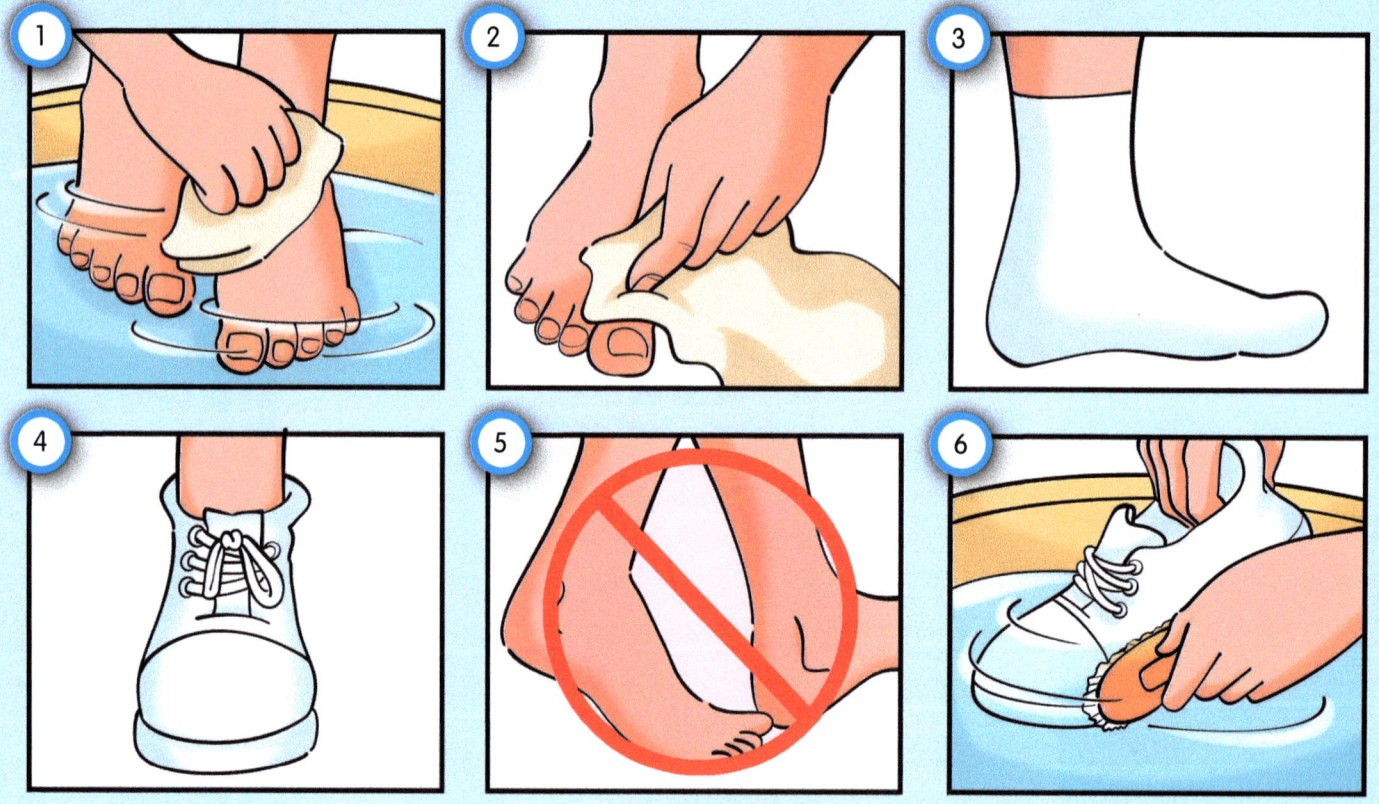

Used water can be collected in pails and basins for flushing the toilet, rinsing the floor of the corridor or, if it's not soapy, for watering plants!

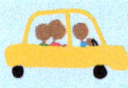 Work with your group again. Use the ball your teacher will give you. The leader starts by throwing the ball to a member of the group. The person who catches the ball will tell the group one of the six things they should do to keep their feet clean.

Too Smart To Start

Lessons 7 & 8

Name: Class: Date:

Hidden in the picture below are eight substances that could be harmful to your health. Can you find and circle them?

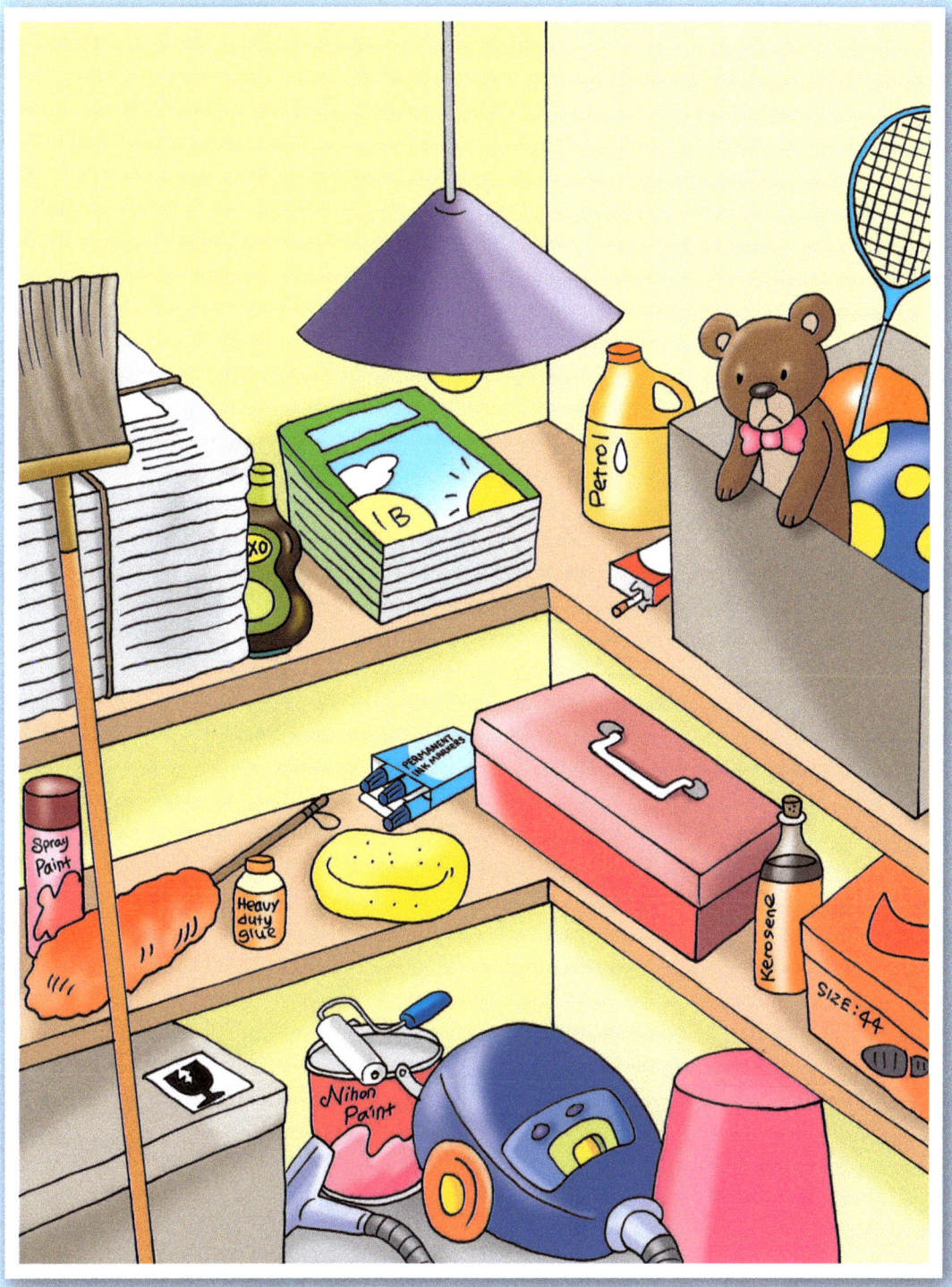

Learning Objective: Pupils will be able to understand how to establish daily habits for caring for their bodies in order to maintain or improve health and prevent illnesses.

The items below are very dangerous because they contain chemicals that are poisonous. They are also very addictive. This means that a person who begins abusing them will find it extremely difficult to stop. Also, long-term use of these substances has harmful effects on the health of the abuser.

Inhalants

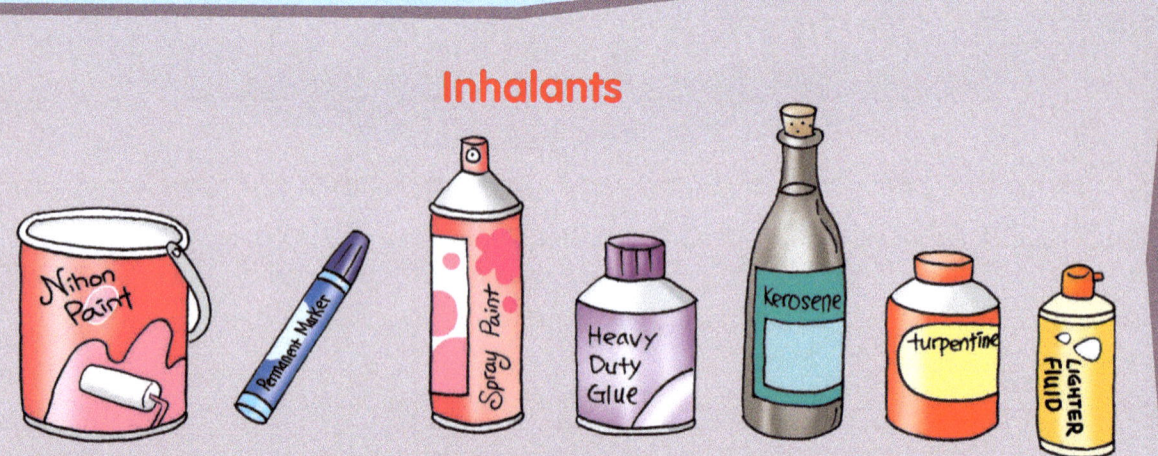

Inhalants are substances that can be commonly found in the home, such as nail polish remover, paint or turpentine, which give off strong-smelling, poisonous gases. Inhaling these gases can cause a bad cough, memory loss, brain damage and death.

Alcohol

Alcohol can cause confusion, loss of coordination and even loss of consciousness. This is why people often meet with accidents on the road after drinking alcohol.

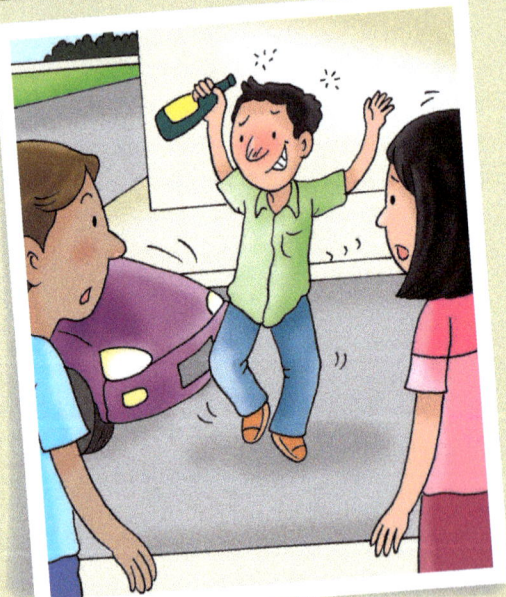

A person who is addicted to alcohol is called an 'alcoholic'. Alcoholics run the risk of liver failure, cancer, heart disease, and brain and nerve damage.

Alcohol is found in 'soda pop', beer, wine and different types of liquor. Underaged drinking is against the law. The legal (allowed by the law) age for drinking and buying alcohol may be different in each country.

In your country, what is the legal age to buy and drink alcohol?

coordination: the control you have over the movements of your body.

Many teenagers smoke, take drugs and sniff glue because they think it makes them look cool and seem more grown up. Others do it because of peer pressure, or to 'escape from their problems'. Unfortunately, these harmful habits only create more problems. They do not know what they are breathing into their lungs.

Below are some ingredients in cigarettes. Do you want these chemicals in your body?

Some ingredients in cigarettes

Nicotine — Main ingredient in insecticide

Carbon monoxide — Dangerous gas from car exhaust

Tar — Sticky substance used to build roads

Naphthalene — Found in mothballs

Hydrogen cyanide — Gas chamber poison

Arsenic — Found in rat poison

Ammonia — Used in floor cleaners

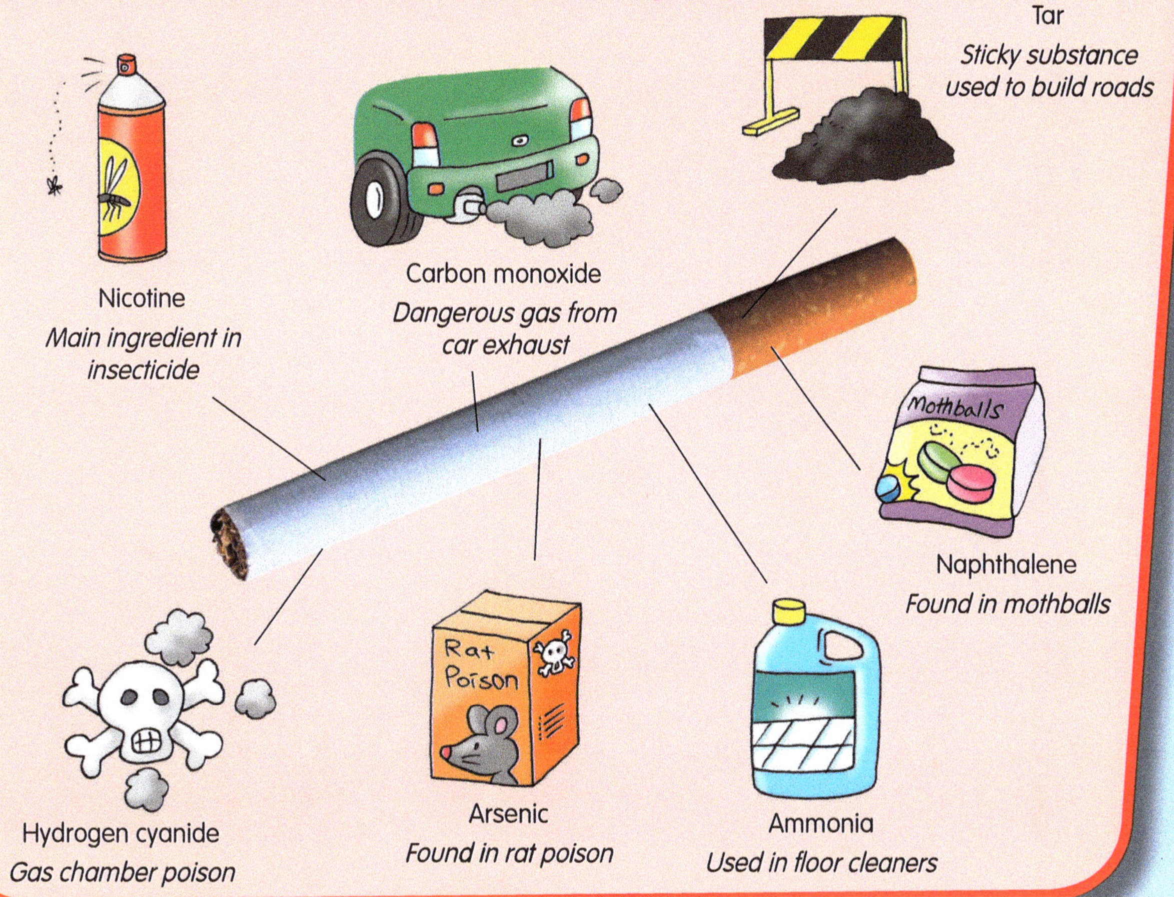

Drugs can kill and cause great harm to your body. Say NO TO DRUGS!

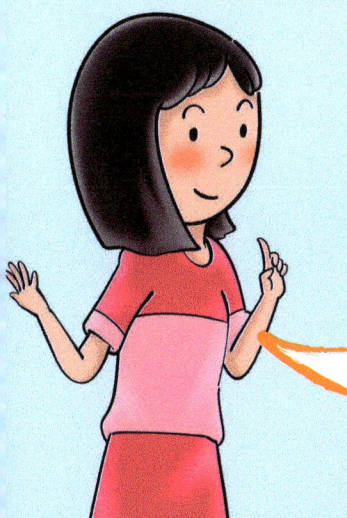

The substances in cigarettes can give you problems in breathing, a bad cough or bad breath. They might also be the cause of cancer, and lung and heart diseases. Some smokers die early too. Now, do you think that's 'cool'?

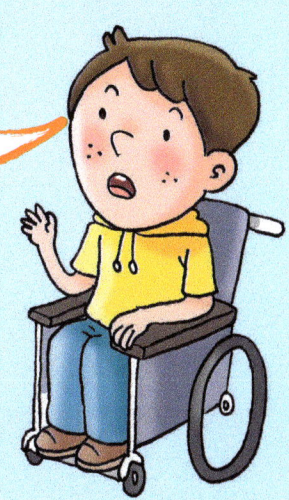

Even if you don't smoke, you can become a 'passive smoker' if you are often around people who smoke. This means you breathe in air which contains cigarette smoke. You too may have the same serious health problems as smokers. Do members in your family smoke? What advice can you give them?

The best way to fight addiction is to never start. If someone asks you to try any harmful substances, just say 'NO!'. Your life and health are worth much more than a few moments of 'fun' and 'excitement'.

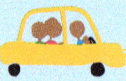 Fill in each speech bubble with what you think the superfriends should say to those offering them harmful substances.

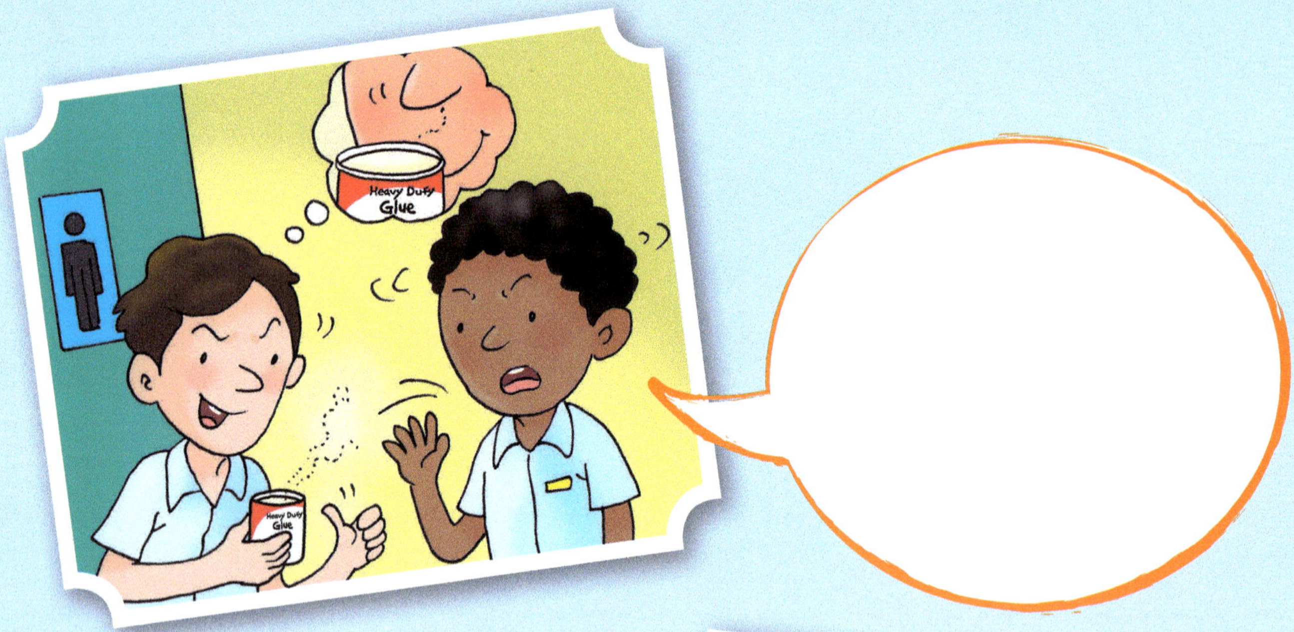

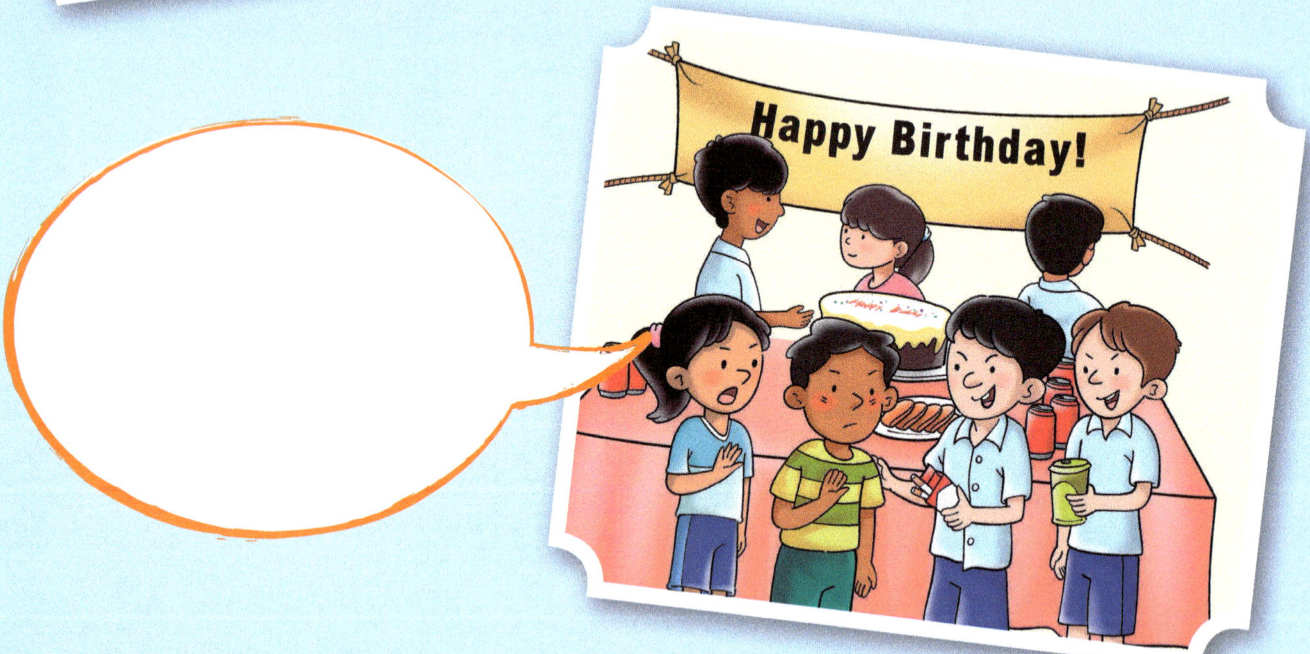

A good way to help you stand firm in your decision to stay addiction-free is to prepare yourself by thinking up and memorising your refusal now. Do not wait for the day someone asks you to take a sniff, puff or gulp before you come up with a reply!

If you know of anyone from your school sharing, buying or selling drugs in school, inform your teacher immediately!

My Precious Sight

Lesson 9

Name: Class: Date:

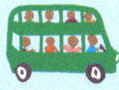 Did you know that myopia, or short-sightedness, is a problem that affects many children and adults in Southeast Asia? If the eyes are not taken care of properly, myopia can become very severe and even lead to loss of sight.

Normal vision

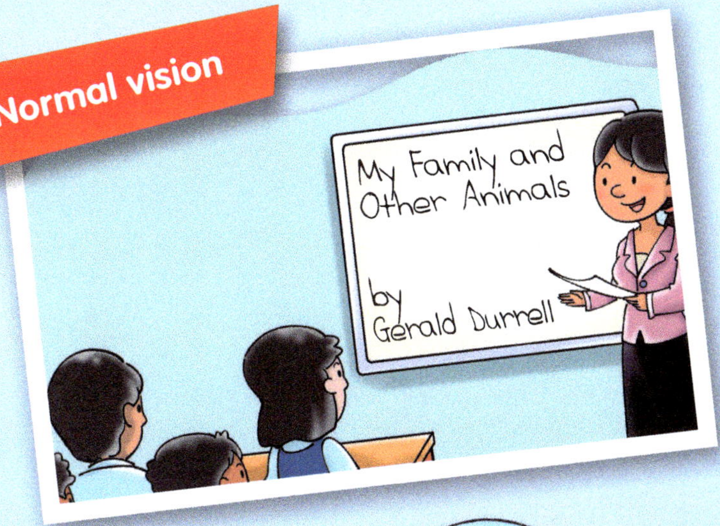

Myopic vision

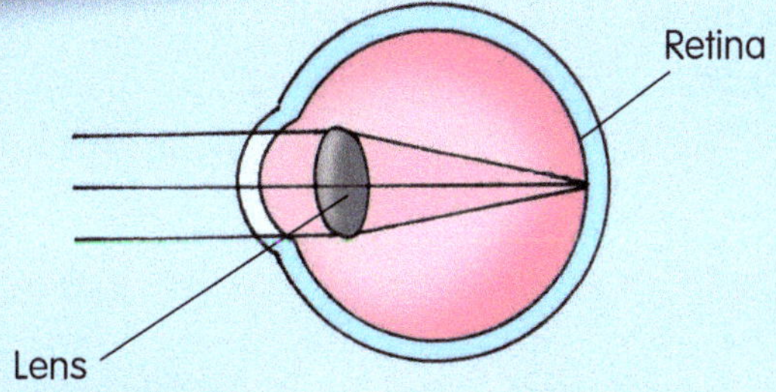

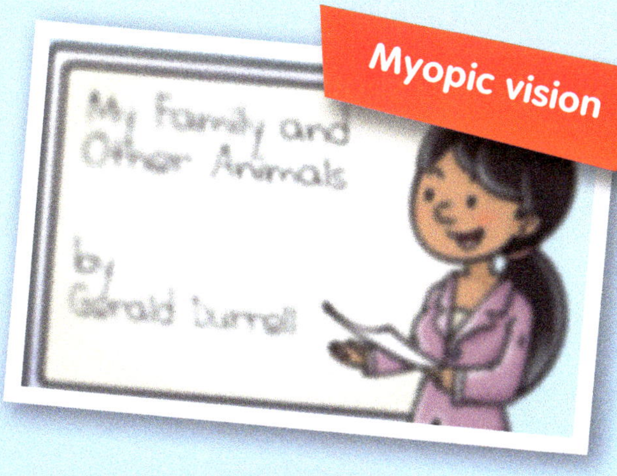

Normal eye

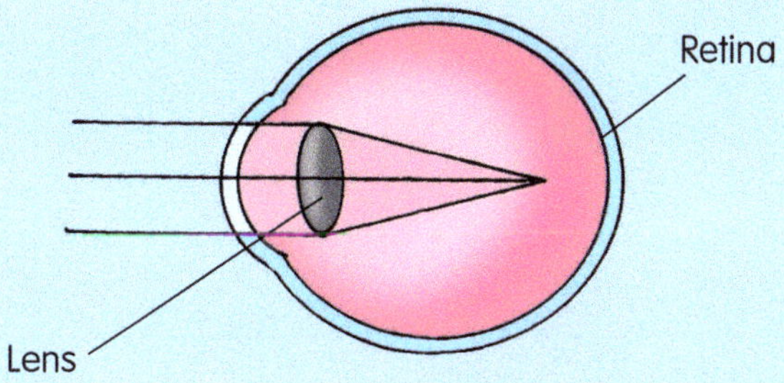

Myopic eye

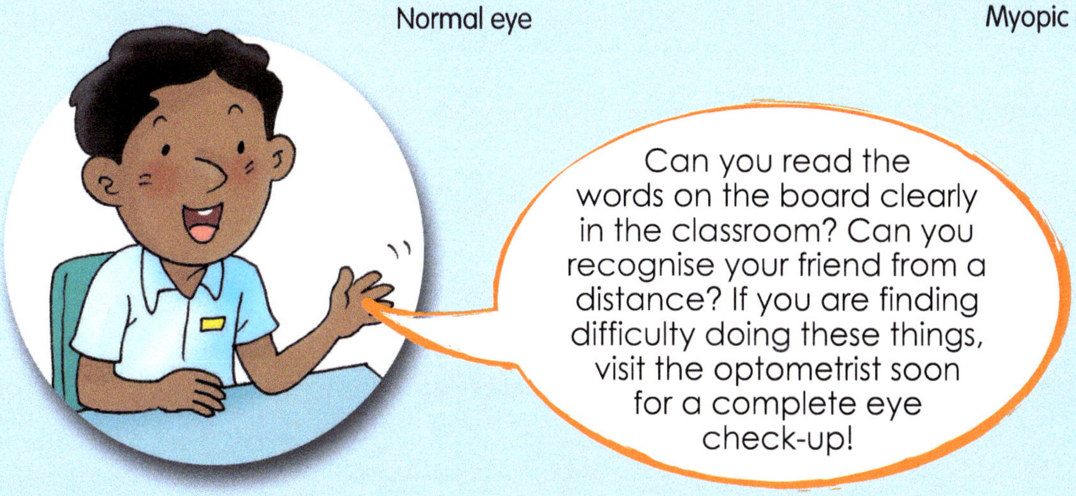

Can you read the words on the board clearly in the classroom? Can you recognise your friend from a distance? If you are finding difficulty doing these things, visit the optometrist soon for a complete eye check-up!

optometrist: an eye care professional who is able to examine your eyes and give you a prescription for spectacles.

Learning Objective: Pupils will be able to recognise that the eyes need proper care and rest for good vision.

There is no cure for myopia, but there are ways you can protect your eyes to prevent the condition from getting worse. Even if you do not have myopia, you should do everything you can to keep your eyes healthy!

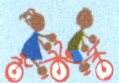 Do you remember how you can protect your eyes? Read each statement below and circle 'T' if it is true and 'F' if it is false.

The Eye Care Quiz

1. You should go for a check-up every year even if you think you can see clearly.   T / F

2. You should limit screen time to less than two hours a day.   T / F

3. You should take a break after about 20 or 30 minutes of near work.   T / F

4. You should read or work in a room with good lighting.   T / F

5. You should sit as close as possible to the TV so that you do not strain your eyes.   T / F

6. Doing some outdoor activities every day is good for your eyes.   T / F

7. Do not stare directly at the sun or any bright light, even if you are wearing sunglasses.   T / F

8. It is not necessary to wear glasses even if you are myopic or short-sighted.   T / F

9. It is all right to lie on your back and read as long as you have your glasses on.   T / F

10. A balanced diet, regular exercise and sufficient sleep will help keep your eyes healthy.   T / F

Name: Class: Date:

Lesson 10

Myopia Or Short-Sightedness

Read the story below.

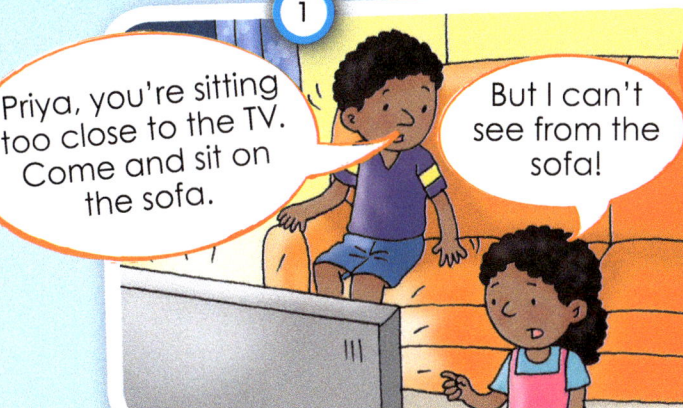

1. "Priya, you're sitting too close to the TV. Come and sit on the sofa."
   "But I can't see from the sofa!"

2. "I missed the bus so many times this week because I couldn't see the number clearly."
   "Oh dear! I'd better ask Mummy to bring you to the optometrist."

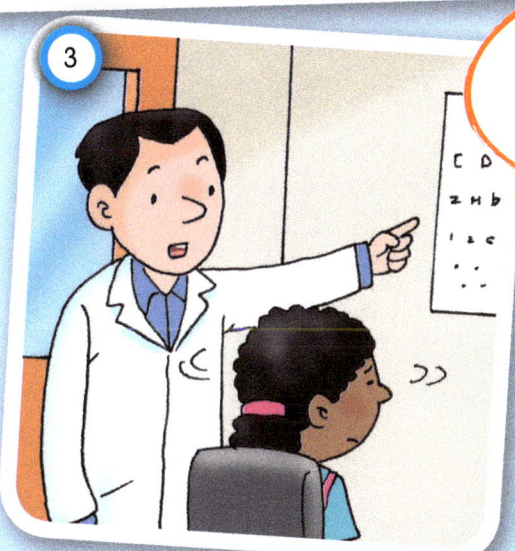

3.

"It looks like Priya has myopia. She needs a pair of glasses."

4.

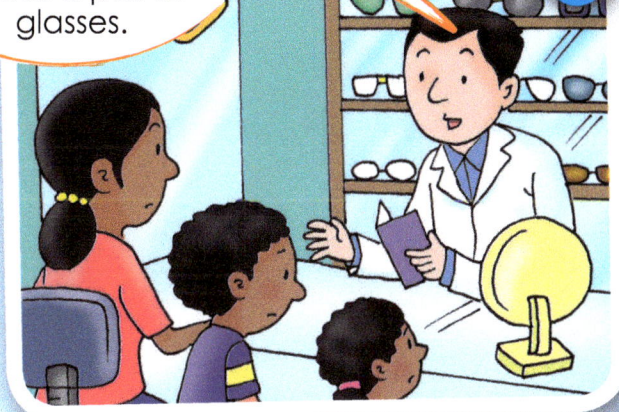

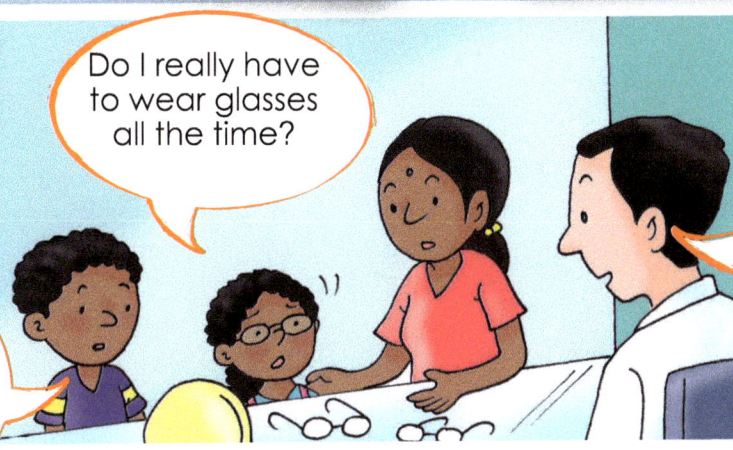

5. "Do I really have to wear glasses all the time?"
   "Yes, Priya. They will help you see better and stop your eyesight from getting worse. Come back next year for a check-up."
   "Don't worry, Priya. You'll get used to it!"

Learning Objective: Pupils will be able to recognise that the eyes need proper care and rest for good vision.

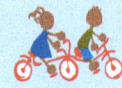 There are many myths about ways to manage myopia. How well can you tell fact from fiction? Write 'fact' in the box for statements that you think are true and 'fiction' for those that you think are false.

1. Wearing spectacles all the time will cause your eyes to become weak because they will rely on the spectacles to help them see. Your eyesight will then get worse.

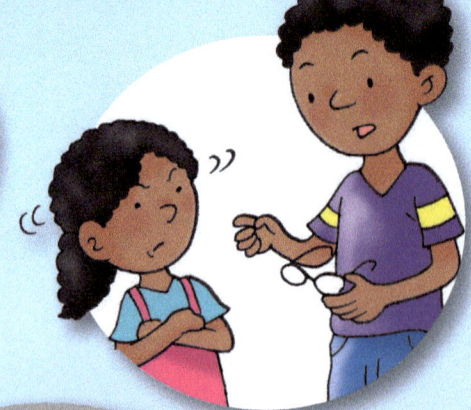

2. Wearing contact lenses helps to reduce myopia by flattening the eyeball. This will make the eyeball shorter so your eyes will be able to focus better.

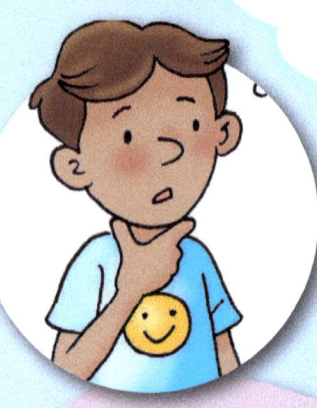

3. Eating food rich in vitamin A will improve myopia.

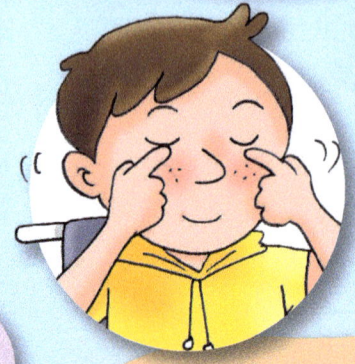

4. Eye exercises and eye massage can help cure myopia.

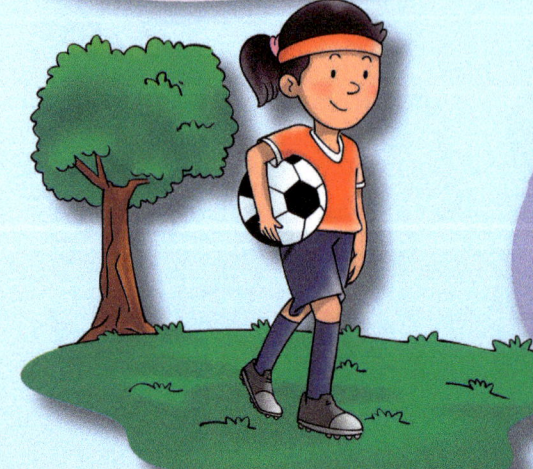

5. Spending some time outdoors every day will give your eyes a rest.

Name: **Class:** **Date:**

Lessons 11 & 12

Do Away With Tooth Decay

You need them to eat, speak and smile. What are they? Your teeth, of course! Life would be difficult without them. Know more about your teeth and take good care of them.

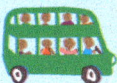 This is a picture of the inside of a tooth. Label the different parts by filling in the blanks with the helping words below.

| pulp | enamel | dentine | gum |

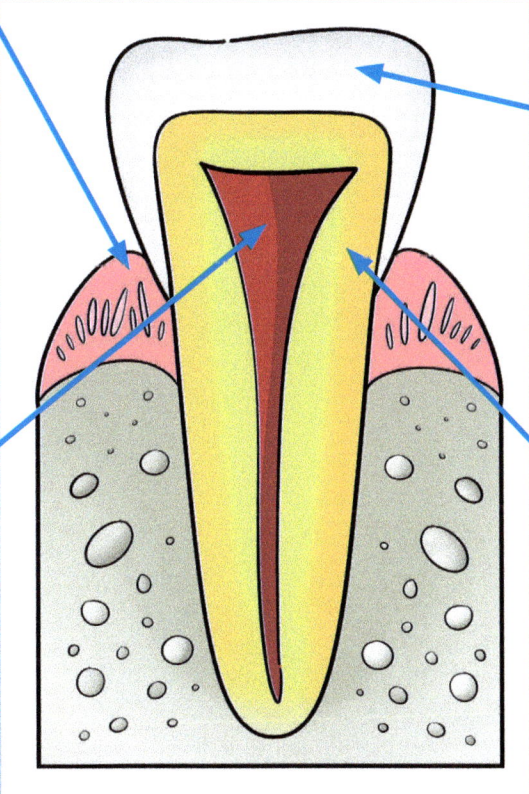

_____
The soft, pink part that holds your teeth in place.

_____
The extremely hard protective outer covering of the tooth.

_____
The innermost part of the tooth. It contains nerves and blood vessels which keep the tooth alive.

_____
The hard, yellow layer that protects the nerves and blood vessels in the tooth.

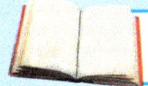 **nerves:** a type of cell in the body that enables you to feel pain or cold.

Learning Objective: Pupils will be able to recognise the importance of developing good oral hygiene habits to ensure that the teeth are well maintained and healthy.

25

Remember to keep your teeth healthy. If you don't, you can develop tooth decay which can unpleasant and painful.

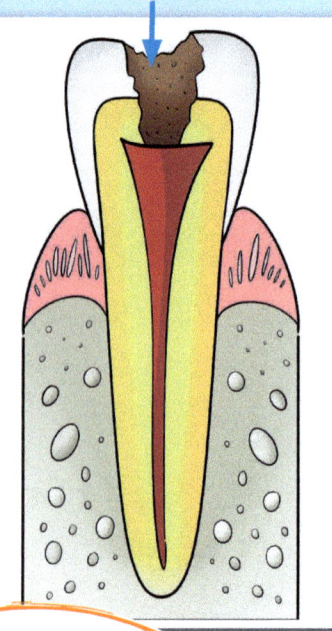
Cavity

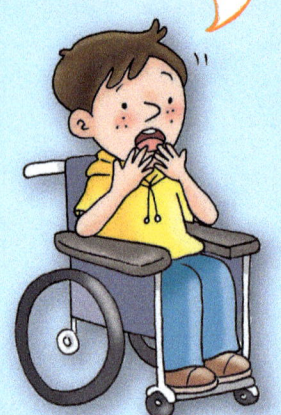
What's tooth decay?

Harold, tooth decay is a disease that is caused by bacteria in the mouth. They act on different types of sugar in food to produce harmful acid. This acid slowly forms a hole in the tooth.

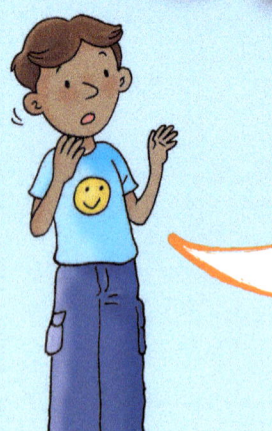
The hole, which dentists call a 'cavity', can create a lot of pain and discomfort. If you don't see a dentist about the decay immediately, you could end up losing your tooth!

The enamel protects the tooth and you should take care of the enamel! Avoid taking fizzy drinks and brushing too hard!

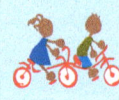 What are some of the warning signs of tooth decay? List down four signs below.

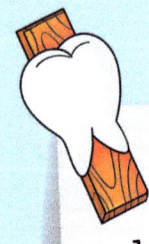

1. _____
2. _____
3. _____
4. _____

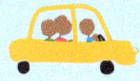 Choose the healthy snacks.

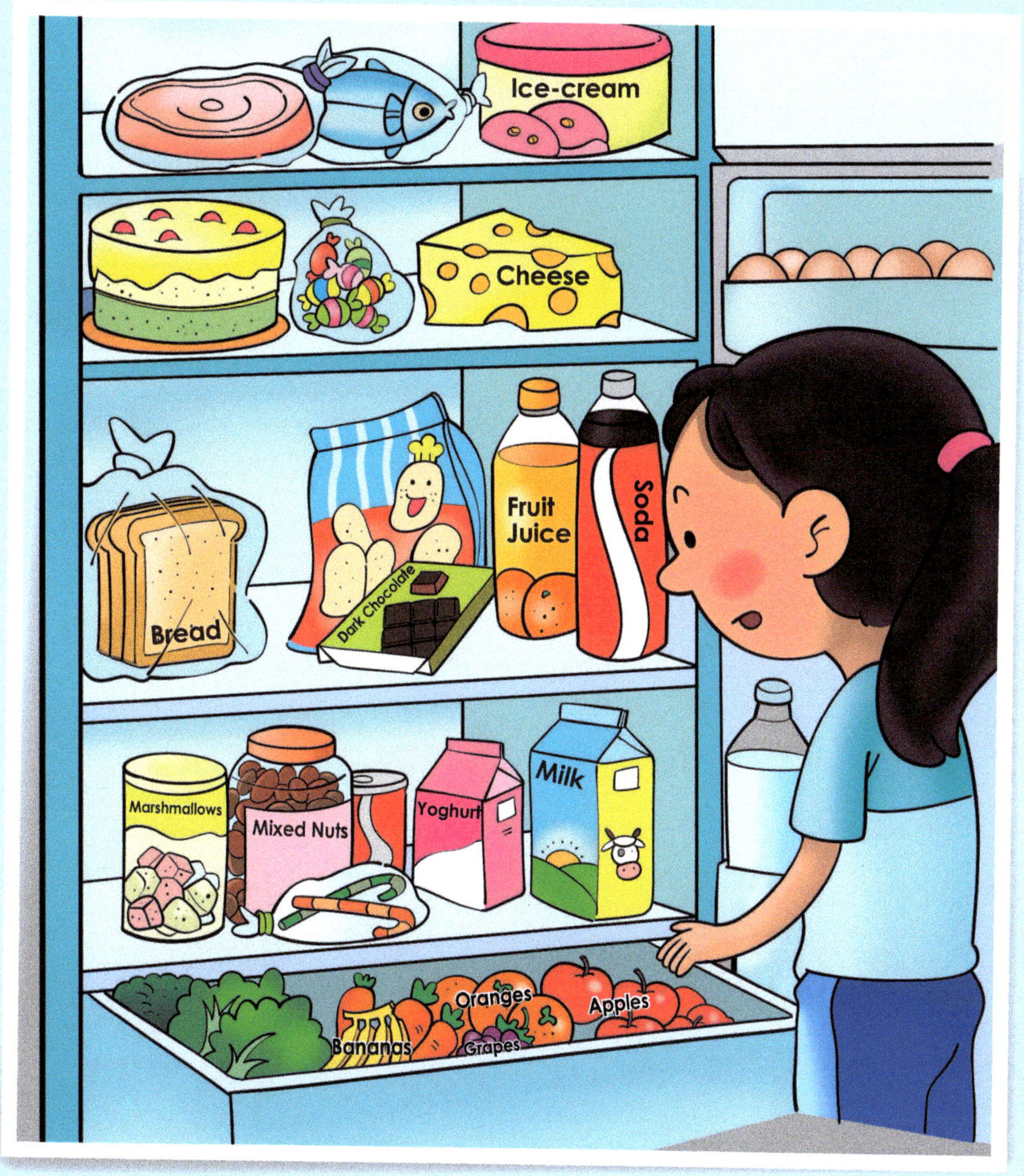

List the healthy snacks: _____

Do you know of other ways in which you can protect your teeth from decay? Fill in the blanks below by using the pictures to help you.

1. B_____ your teeth with f_____ toothpaste at least twice a day—once in the morning and once before you go to b____ at night.

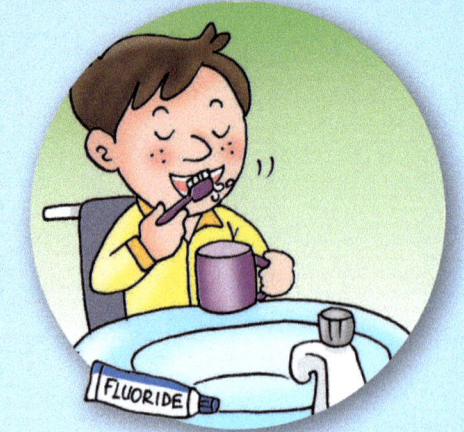

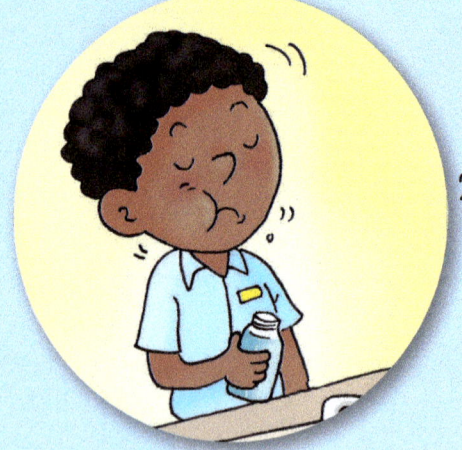

2. R_____ your mouth thoroughly after eating.

3. Use an oral pick or f_____ your teeth after a meal to remove the bits of f_____ that are stuck between your teeth.

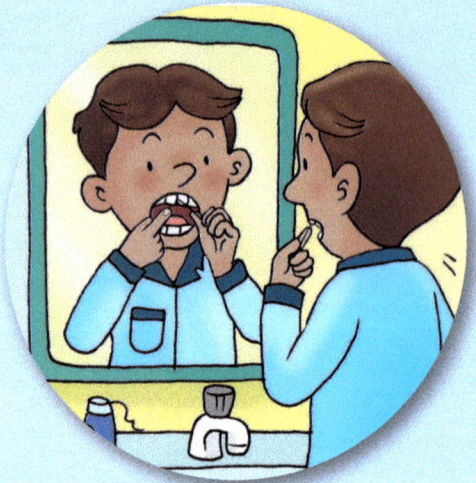

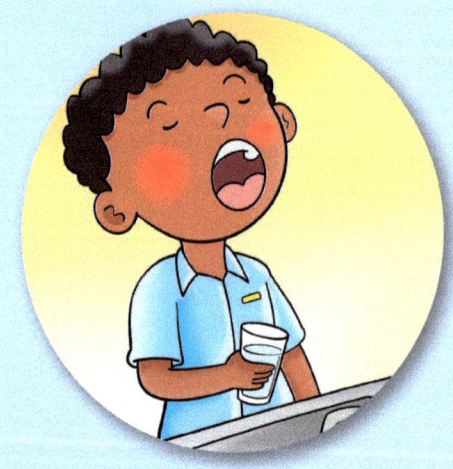

4. G_____ your throat once or twice daily. You can do this with salt water or a mouthwash.

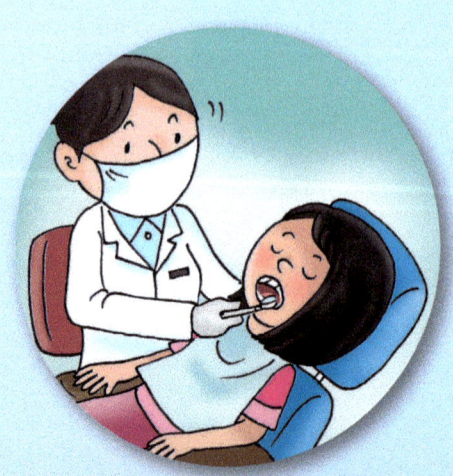

5. Visit the d_____ regularly to check for signs of tooth decay and to remove plaque.

Environment And Your Health

In this section, you will learn about:
- water safety;
- fire safety; and
- food safety.

Being Wise About Water

Lesson 1

Name: ⬜ Class: ⬜ Date: ⬜

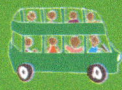 Look at the pictures below. What are the superfriends doing incorrectly?

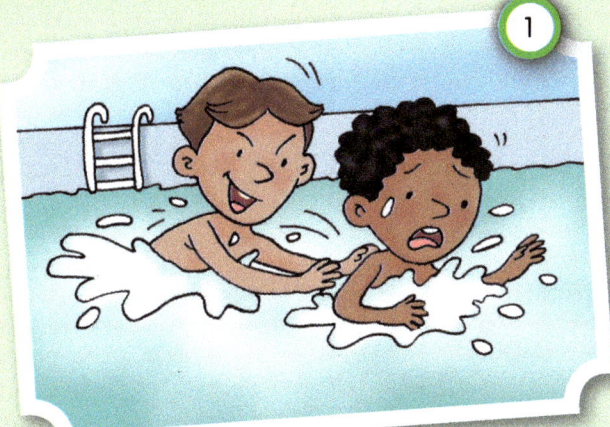

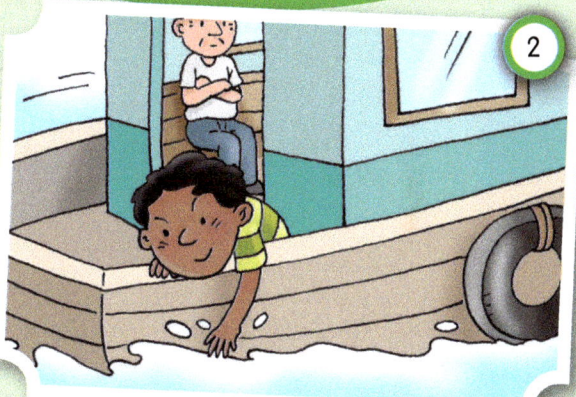

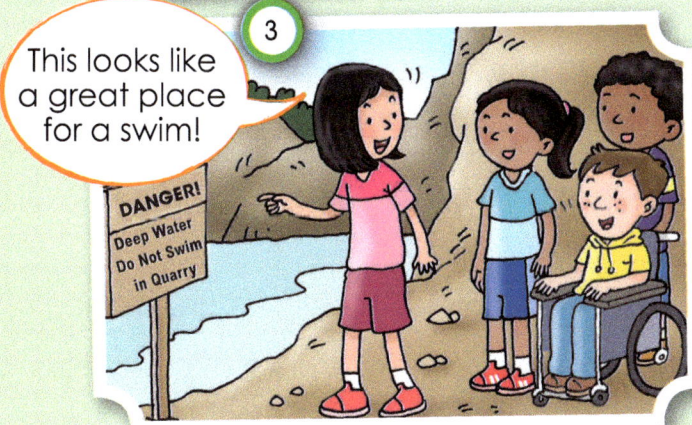

"This looks like a great place for a swim!"

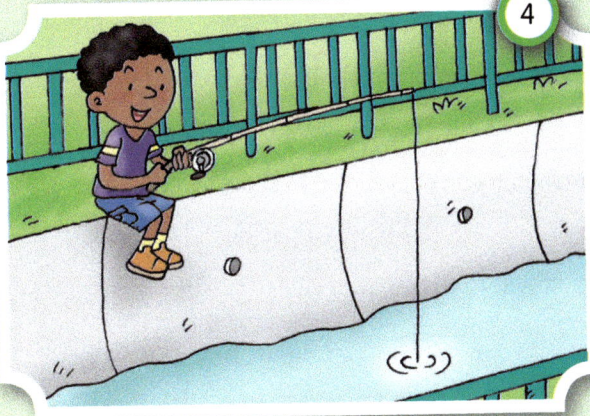

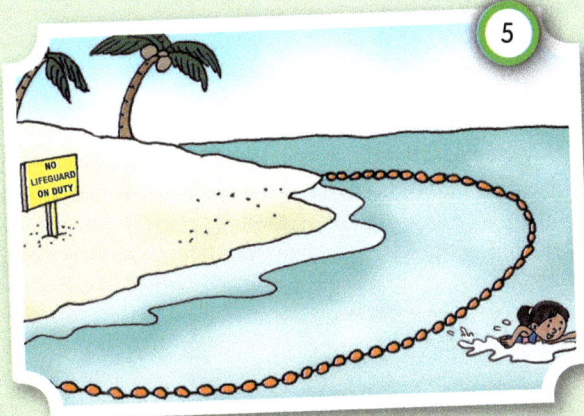

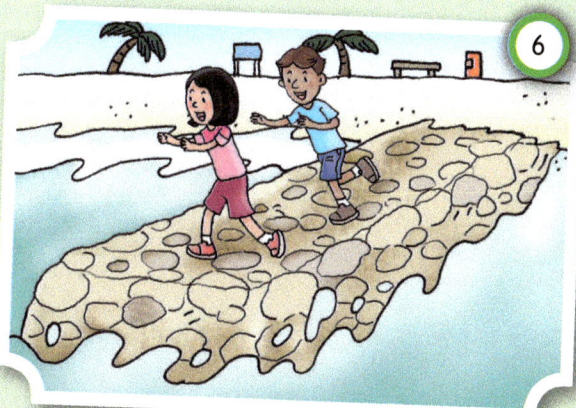

Learning Objective: Pupils will be able to understand that it is everyone's responsibility to keep safe by paying attention to environmental dangers, and recognise that accidents and unsafe situations can occur in school, at home or in unexpected places and circumstances.

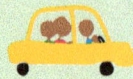 Write down each superfriend's action and say why it is dangerous.

	Action	Why it is dangerous
1.		
2.		
3.		
4.		
5.		
6.		

- Accidents in water can be prevented if you see the danger and follow safety rules.
- Swimming without lifeguards means that if you should have problems in water, there is no one properly trained to help you.
- It is dangerous to swim outside permitted areas (where the risks are higher).
- When fishing or travelling in a small boat on the river, be aware of crocodiles or dangerous creatures (e.g. do not leave your hands or feet in the water).

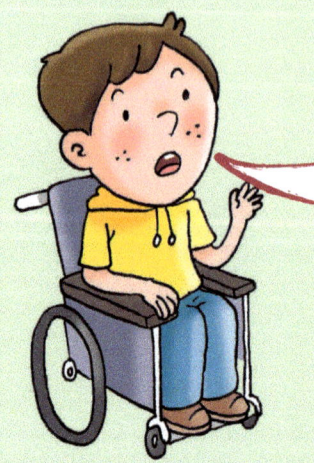

When in water, follow safety rules strictly. Accidents can be prevented. Remember: You are responsible for your own safety!

Name: Class: Date: **Lesson 2**

Dangerous Water

Read the following article and answer the questions that follow on the next page.

Know the Danger Zones and Learn Survival Skills

By Laura Low

"Young people need to understand danger and learn survival skills in open water," said Mr John Lim, Minister of Education, who was attending the wake of Muhammad Alfian, the 11-year-old who drowned off East Coast Park on Tuesday. "Schools need to teach water survival skills, not only because of this tragic incident, but because it's a very useful life skill," the Minister said.

After a two-hour search operation, Alfian's body was found near Bedok Jetty on Tuesday afternoon. Alfian had gone to the beach with friends after finishing a school examination that morning. A 60-year-old swimmer said the four boys were about 40 metres away from the shore when they started to shout for help. The courageous man swam to them and started bringing each back to shore. Alfian had disappeared by the time the man went back to rescue the third boy.

Alfian's uncle and eldest brother told reporters that the Primary 5 pupil did not know how to swim. Even though he had gone through compulsory lessons two years ago, Alfian and a few other pupils could not swim, his former classmates confirmed.

Mr Lim said, "When you're young, you feel safe when you are in a group and you think nothing will go wrong. If you're alone, you may not do it. But in a group, people just jump in."

Simply learning swimming strokes may not be enough when dealing with more difficult situations such as swimming in the sea, said former national swimmer Joseph Wee who is now a swimming instructor. "The water may suddenly appear too deep and strong currents can cause panic and shock when people are not prepared for danger. We can't see what is under the water, especially the water in Singapore, which is not clear."

Earlier in the day, Alfian's father and two older brothers, aged 16 and 19, arrived at the mortuary to collect his body. They left filled with sadness.

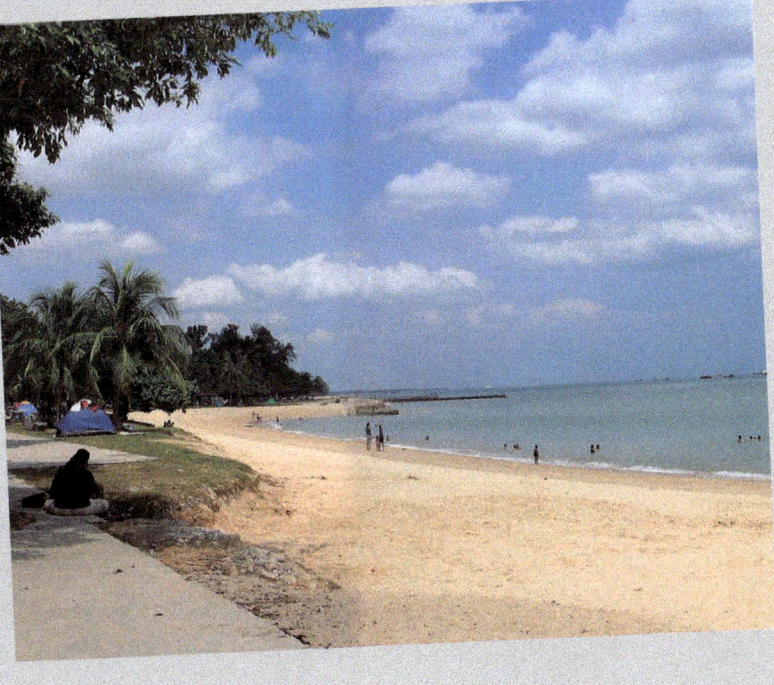

Learning Objective: Pupils will be able to understand that it is everyone's responsibility to keep safe by paying attention to environmental dangers, and recognise that accidents and unsafe situations can occur in school, at home or in unexpected places and circumstances.

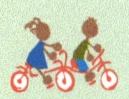 Discuss the following questions with your partner. After your discussion, write the answers down.

1. What are the dangers in swimming in an open sea?
   _____
   _____

2. Why do you think the accident happened?
   _____
   _____

3. Are there water bodies around you? Name them.
   _____
   _____

4. Would you go swimming in the sea or river in a group? Why or why not?
   _____
   _____

5. Write down two important lessons about water safety you have learnt from the article.
   _____
   _____

water body: any area where there is a significant volume of water, such as the sea, ponds, canals, lakes, reservoirs or swimming pools.

Safety At The Pool

Swimming is fun but we need to observe some basic rules at the pool. If you don't follow the rules, you can annoy others or even put yourself in danger.

Haris is at the pool. Go through each picture and write down what Haris should do in each situation.

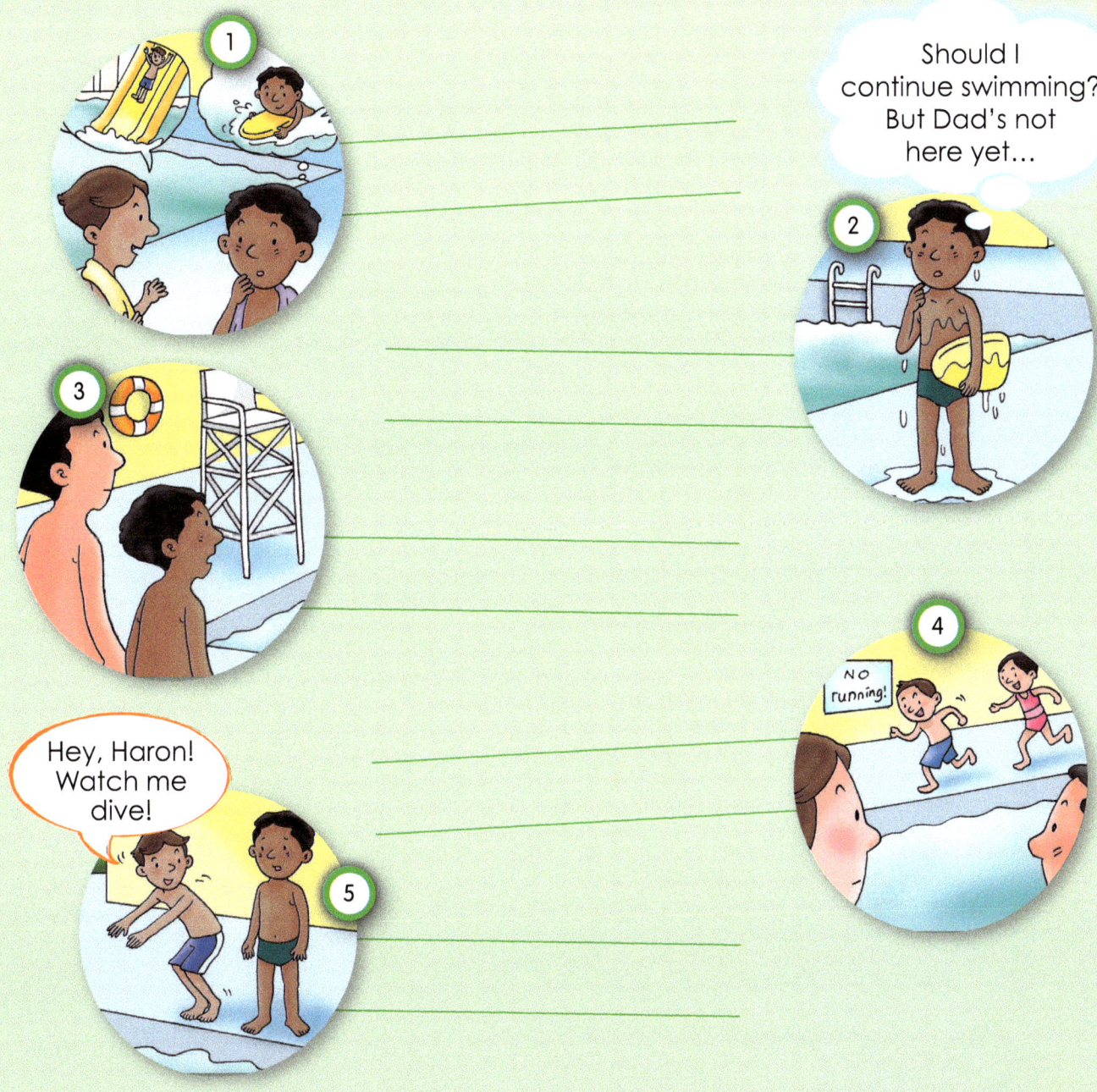

Learning Objective: Pupils will be able to understand that it is everyone's responsibility to keep safe by paying attention to environmental dangers, and recognise that accidents and unsafe situations can occur in school, at home or in unexpected places and circumstances.

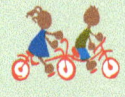 Accidents at the pool can be prevented if everyone follows safety rules. Haris's sister Siti wants to go for a swim in the afternoon. Haris is writing her a note to remind her of the safety rules. Help him complete the note by writing in the spaces below.

Dear Siti,

Please remember these safety rules when you're at the pool later:

1. _____
   _____

2. _____
   _____

3. _____
   _____

4. _____
   _____

5. _____
   _____

Please be careful!

Love, Haris

Name: **Class:** **Date:**

Lesson 4

Fire Hazards In The Home

 Common fire hazards can be found in the home. The picture shows Lam's home and five objects that could start a fire. Circle them and complete the exercise on the next page.

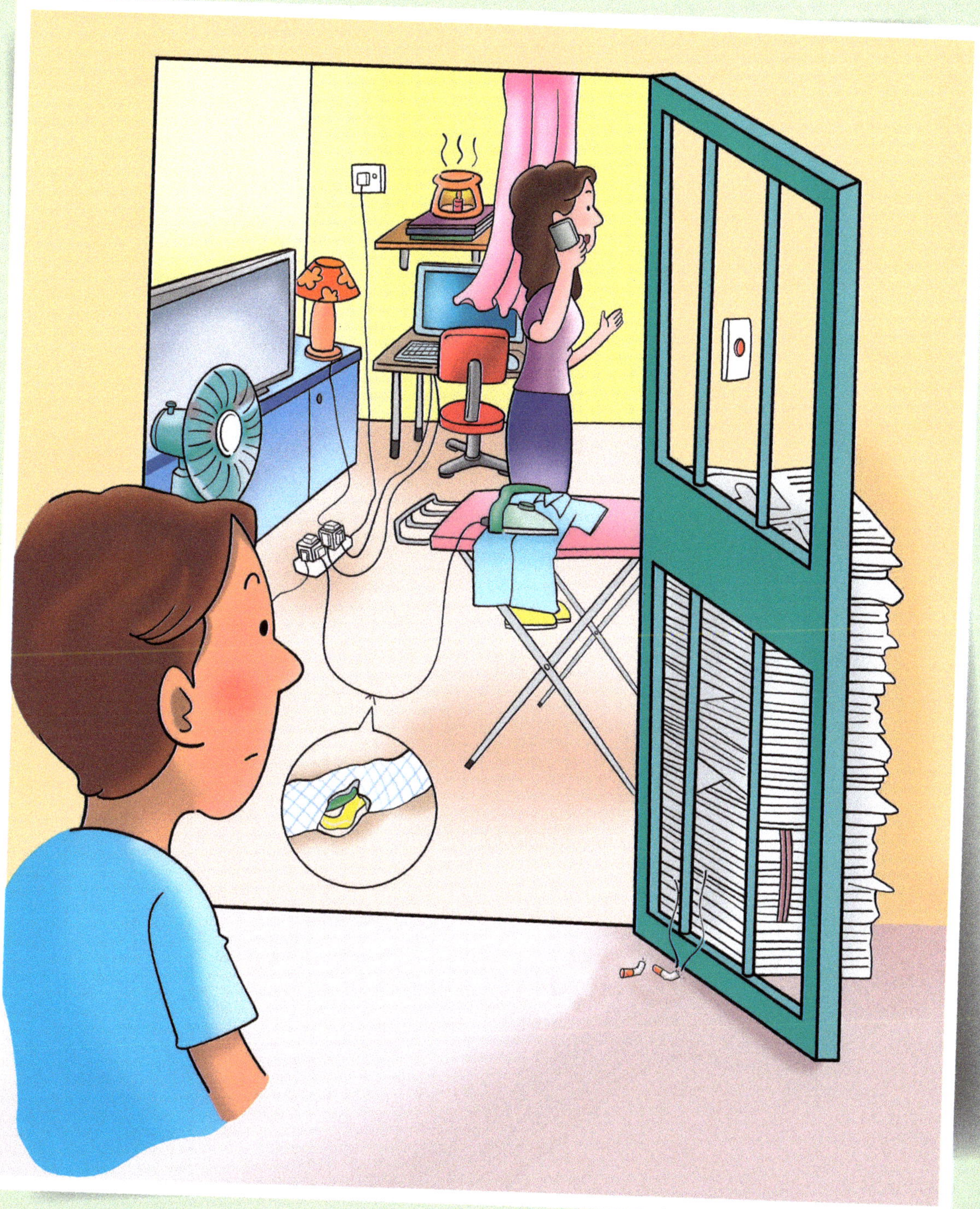

Learning Objective: Pupils will be able to understand that it is everyone's responsibility to keep safe by paying attention to environmental dangers, and recognise that accidents and unsafe situations can occur in school, at home or in unexpected places and circumstances.

37

 Describe each of the five fire hazards and think about how they can be prevented. Write your answers in the spaces below.

Hazard 1

_____

_____

_____

Prevention

_____

_____

_____

Hazard 2

_____

_____

_____

Prevention

_____

_____

_____

Hazard 3

_____

_____

_____

Prevention

_____

_____

_____

Hazard 4

_____

_____

_____

Prevention

_____

_____

_____

Hazard 5

_____

_____

_____

Prevention

_____

_____

_____

Lesson 5

Is Your Home Fire-Safe?

 Harold, Ajit, Eileen and Tawan paid a visit to the neighbourhood fire station. They learnt some simple ways to keep their homes free of fire hazards. What do you think they learnt? Fill in the blanks below.

T _ _ _ _ o_ _ all electrical appliances and un _ _ _ _ them if you are not using them.

Make sure there are enough electrical outlets. Do not _ _ _ _ load a socket.
Plugging in too many electrical appliances can cause overheating. This is a common cause of fires in the home.

Always keep matches, lighters and candles in a _ _ _ _ place, away from children.
Throw away flammable objects in a _ _ _ _ area too. One example is old n _ _ _ _ _ _ _ _ _. Avoid leaving them at the corridor where someone might throw out a c _ _ _ _ _ _ _ _ butt.

Do not leave a f _ _ _ burning without paying attention to it.
Having a f _ _ _ e _ _ _ _ _ _ _ _ _ _ is helpful too. It could save lives.

Learning Objective: Pupils will be able to understand that it is everyone's responsibility to keep safe by paying attention to environmental dangers, and recognise dangerous situations and react to them in ways to reduce any harmful effects.

39

It is not hard to keep your home safe from fire hazards. You just need to be aware and alert to the possible dangers in your home.

In each space below, describe each fire hazard you have 'observed' from your walkthrough of your home. Then, write what actions can be taken to prevent a fire.

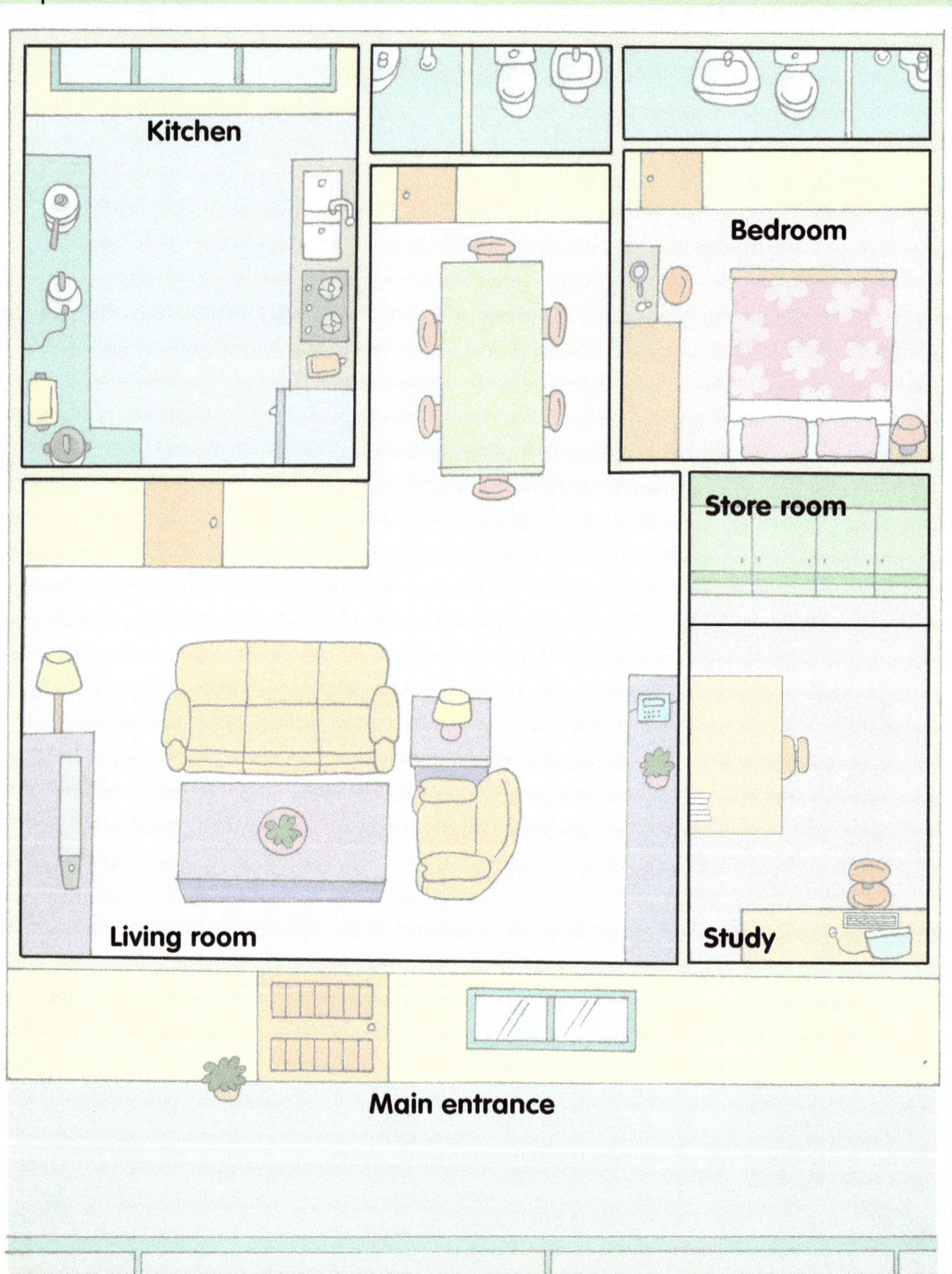

Name: **Class:** **Date:**

Lesson 6

Fire Strikes

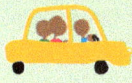 Play this game in your group. You will need a dice and some counters. Start at 1 and end exactly at 30.

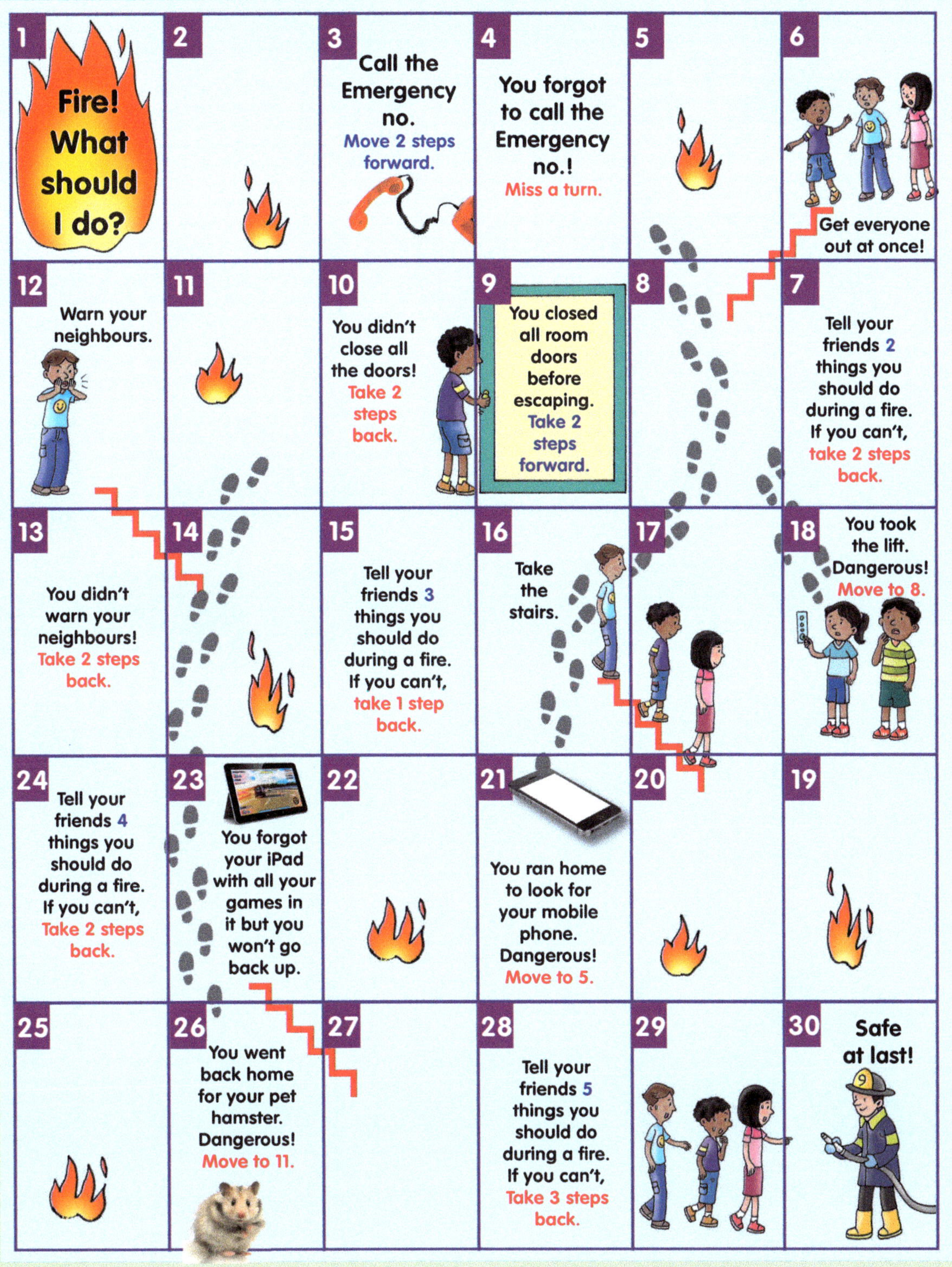

1 Fire! What should I do?	2	3 Call the Emergency no. Move 2 steps forward.	4 You forgot to call the Emergency no.! Miss a turn.	5	6 Get everyone out at once!
12 Warn your neighbours.	11	10 You didn't close all the doors! Take 2 steps back.	9 You closed all room doors before escaping. Take 2 steps forward.	8	7 Tell your friends 2 things you should do during a fire. If you can't, take 2 steps back.
13 You didn't warn your neighbours! Take 2 steps back.	14	15 Tell your friends 3 things you should do during a fire. If you can't, take 1 step back.	16 Take the stairs.	17	18 You took the lift. Dangerous! Move to 8.
24 Tell your friends 4 things you should do during a fire. If you can't, Take 2 steps back.	23 You forgot your iPad with all your games in it but you won't go back up.	22	21 You ran home to look for your mobile phone. Dangerous! Move to 5.	20	19
25	26 You went back home for your pet hamster. Dangerous! Move to 11.	27	28 Tell your friends 5 things you should do during a fire. If you can't, Take 3 steps back.	29	30 Safe at last!

Learning Objective: Pupils will be able to recognise dangerous situations and react to them in ways to reduce any harmful effects.

41

In a fire, the smoke is thick and dark. That makes it very difficult for a person to see anything. The smoke also gives out different types of poisonous gas that can kill you. So if you are caught in a fire, it is very important that you search for clean air.

 What are the correct actions to take if you are in a room filled with smoke from a fire?

Describe what you should do:

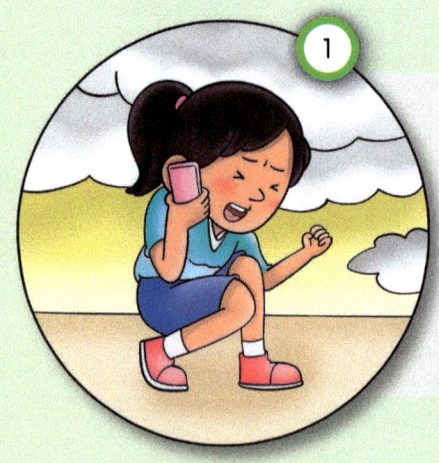

1

What number do you call to report a fire in your country?

_____
_____
_____

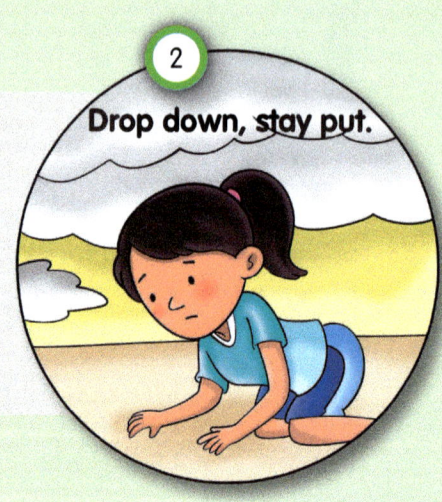

2

Drop down, stay put.

_____
_____
_____

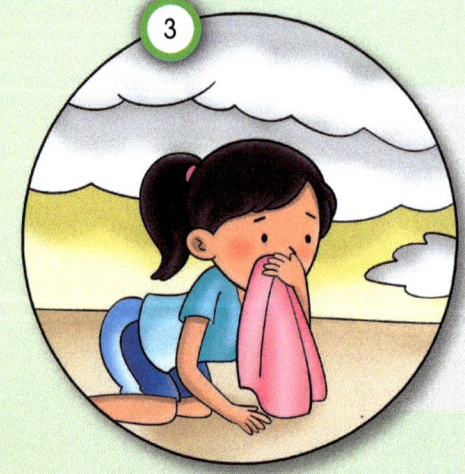

3

_____
_____
_____

emits: gives out.

Name: Class: Date:

Lesson 7

What's In Your Food?

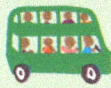 Haris has just recovered from food poisoning. Because he never wants it to happen again, he needs to find out more about it and how he can prevent it. Read the information he has found.

Food poisoning

Food poisoning is caused by eating food that contains germs such as harmful bacteria. Bacteria are living things that are so tiny they can only be seen through a microscope. Even though you can't see them, bacteria are everywhere! They can be found on flies, faeces, toilets, computer keyboards, and unclean surfaces. If they get onto your food, you can become very ill.

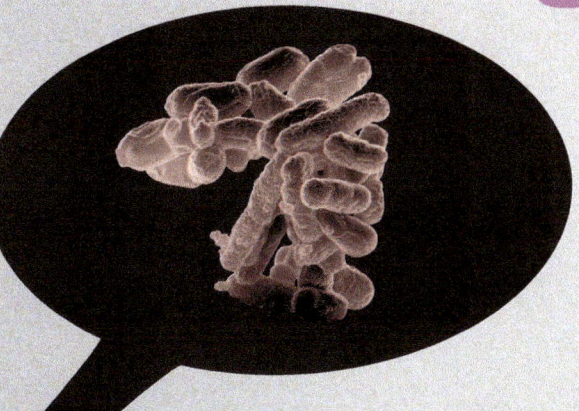

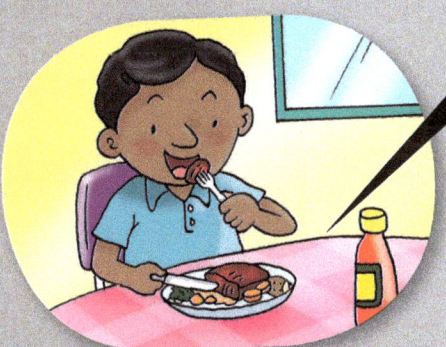

If you do not want to get food poisoning, make sure your food does not become contaminated. Avoid food that is raw or half-cooked. Eat food that is properly cooked and keep it covered if you are not ready to eat it. Practise good hygiene habits and wash your hands and utensils well before starting a meal.

When you are down with food poisoning, you may experience fever, diarrhoea, vomiting and stomach pain. This usually lasts for a short while but in more serious cases, you can be ill for weeks.

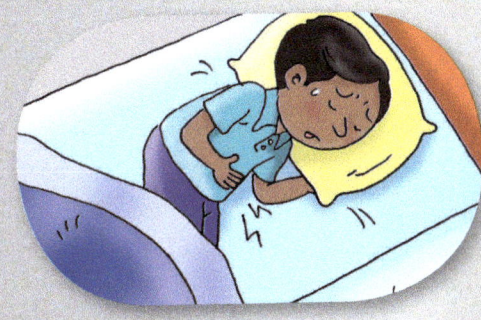

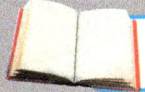 **contaminated:** something that is made dirty because of a harmful substance.

Learning Objective: Pupils will be able to recognise that an unclean environment is a risk to healthy living for everyone.

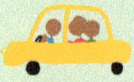

Haris wants to find out what caused his food poisoning. Help him solve the mystery by cracking the secret code below. Then write out the hidden message.

6 – 3 – 9 – 60 – 15 – 54 – 27 – 3
gives you
B   A   C   T   E   R   I   A

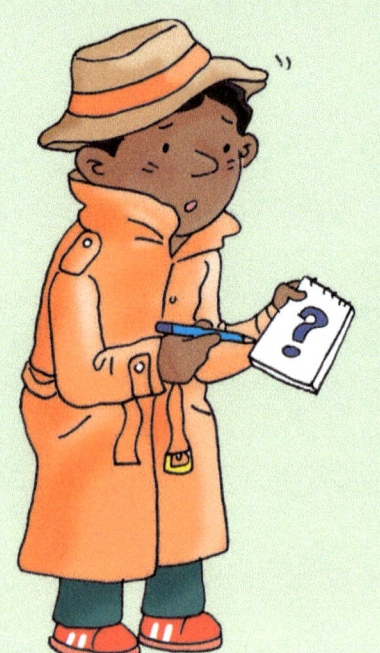

24-15   12-27-12

42-45-60   69-3-57-24

24-27-57   24-3-42-12-57

3-18-60-15-54   21-45-27-42-21

60-45   60-24-15

60-45-27-36-15-60

Haris had food poisoning because _____

_____

_____

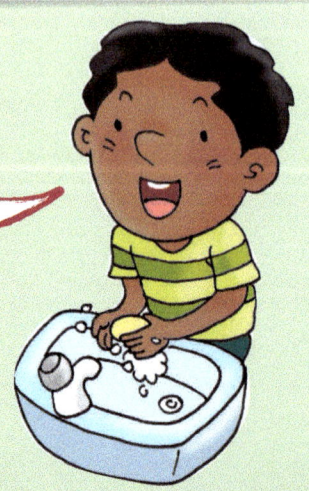

Bacteria can be found everywhere. Practise good hygiene habits so that you don't spread germs to the food you eat.

Name: Class: Date:

Lesson 8

Practise Good Food Hygiene

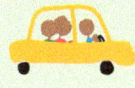 Look at the following pictures. Discuss in your group the mistake each superfriend is making.

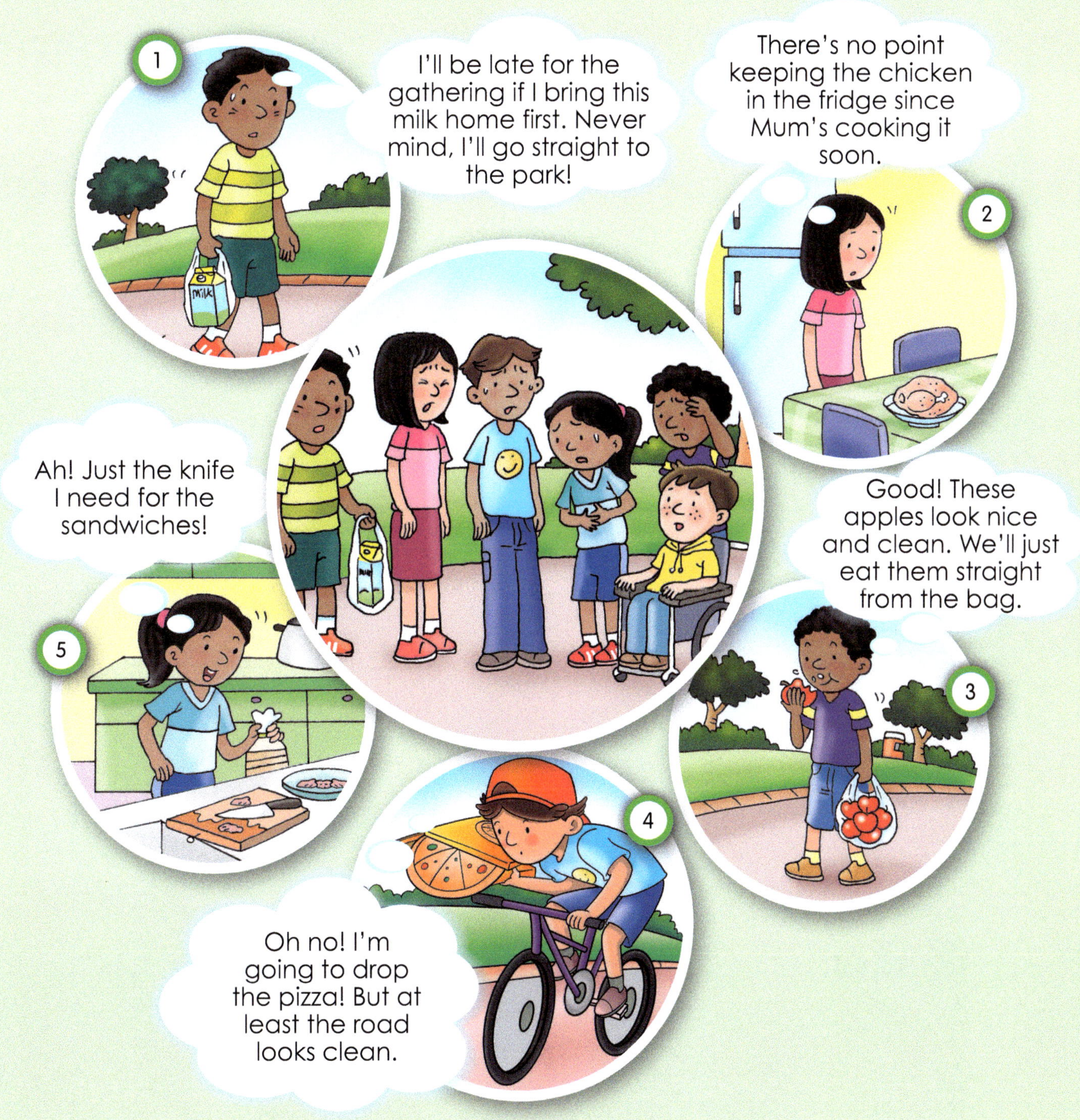

1 I'll be late for the gathering if I bring this milk home first. Never mind, I'll go straight to the park!

2 There's no point keeping the chicken in the fridge since Mum's cooking it soon.

5 Ah! Just the knife I need for the sandwiches!

3 Good! These apples look nice and clean. We'll just eat them straight from the bag.

4 Oh no! I'm going to drop the pizza! But at least the road looks clean.

Learning Objective: Pupils will be able to recognise that an unclean environment is a risk to healthy living for everyone.

45

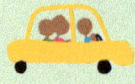

Describe the mistake made by each superfriend in the column under 'Mistake'. In the last column, explain why it was unsafe and what each should have done to practise good food hygiene.

	Mistake	Why it is unsafe and what should have been done
1. Haris		
2. Eileen		
3. Ajit		
4. Lam		
5. Tawan		

46

Lesson 9

Let's Practise Food Safety

 Haris, Tawan and Ajit have volunteered to operate a food stall at their school's fundraiser event. They will be making sandwiches. However, not everything seems right! Imagine you are a health inspector from the Ministry of Environment. Can you spot and circle at least eight unhygienic practices?

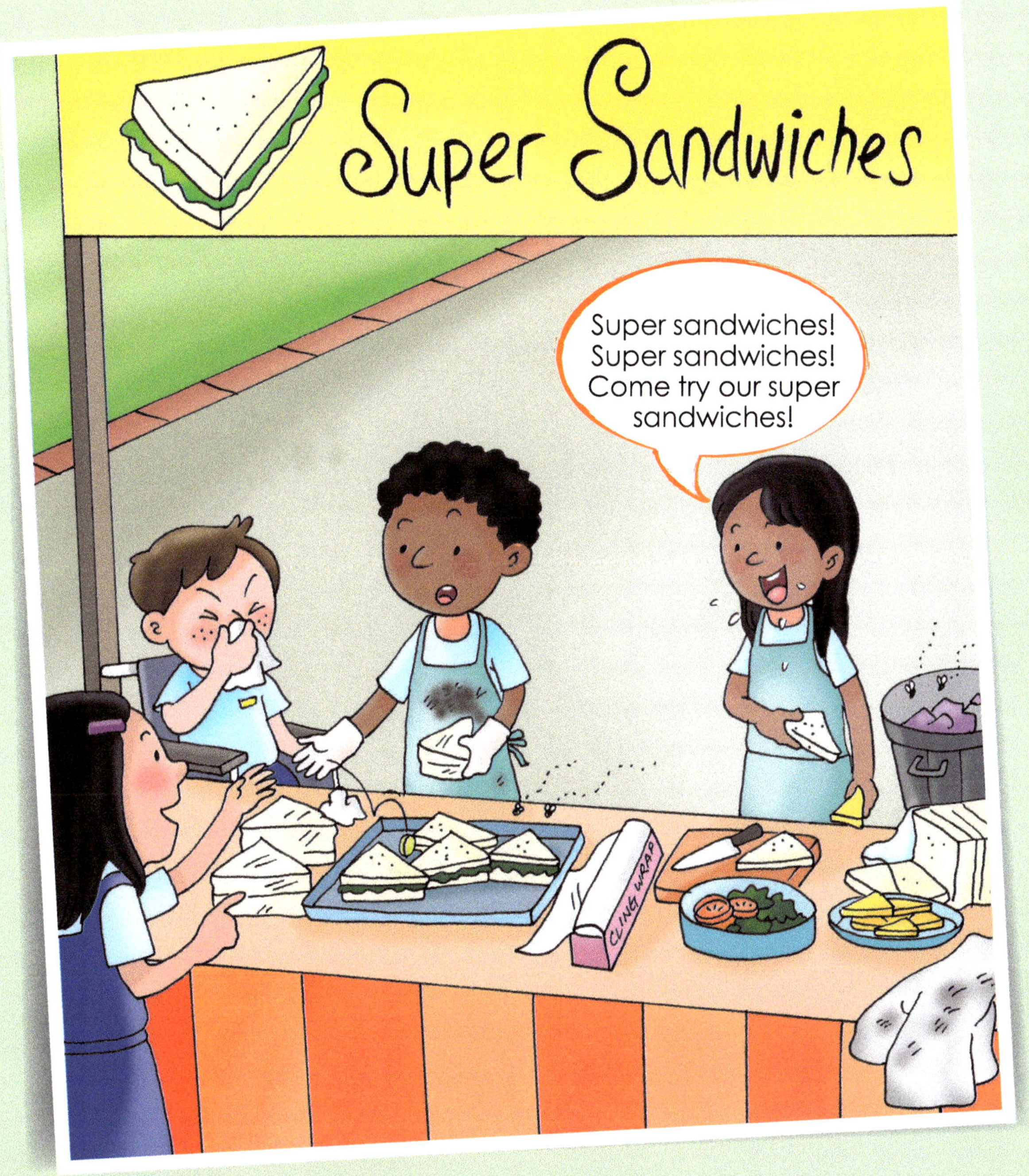

Learning Objective: Pupils will be able to recognise that an unclean environment is a risk to healthy living for everyone.

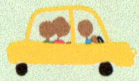

The school wants to carry out a survey of the hygiene practices of its canteen vendors. Your help as a health inspector is needed! Come up with six more questions for the survey below. The first two have been done as examples for you.

Good Hygiene Practices Survey

1. Are there any stalls where there are flies?   Yes / No

2. Are there any vendors in the canteen who do not wear gloves when handling food?   Yes / No

3. _____   Yes / No

4. _____   Yes / No

5. _____   Yes / No

6. _____   Yes / No

7. _____   Yes / No

8. _____   Yes / No

Emotional And Psychological Health

In this section, you will learn:

- the importance of self-confidence; and
- how to protect yourself from abuse.

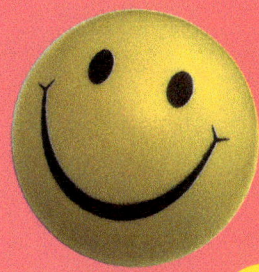

Name:　　　　　　　　Class:　　　　Date:

Lesson 1

Building My Confidence

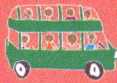 Look at the pictures below. Haris, Tawan and Ajit do not feel good about themselves. Why do you think they are feeling this way?

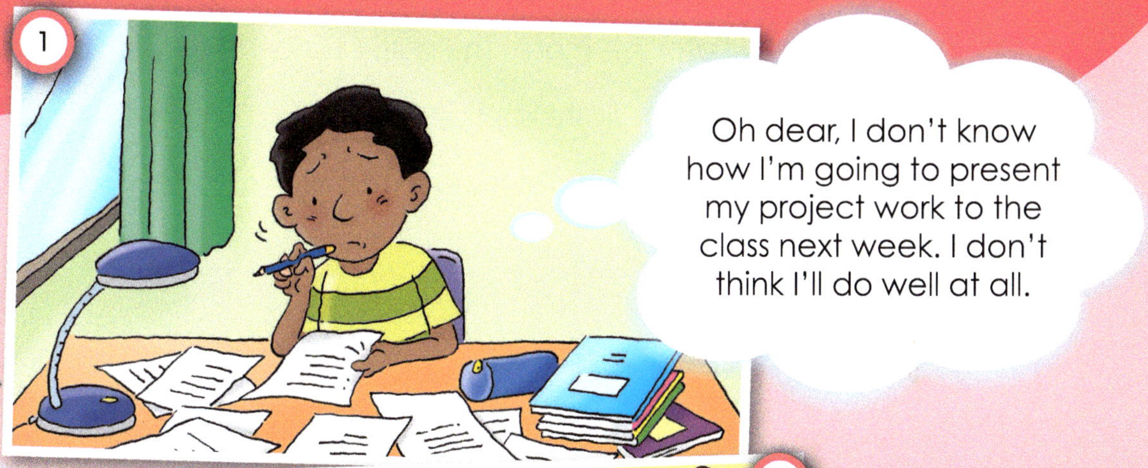

1. *Oh dear, I don't know how I'm going to present my project work to the class next week. I don't think I'll do well at all.*

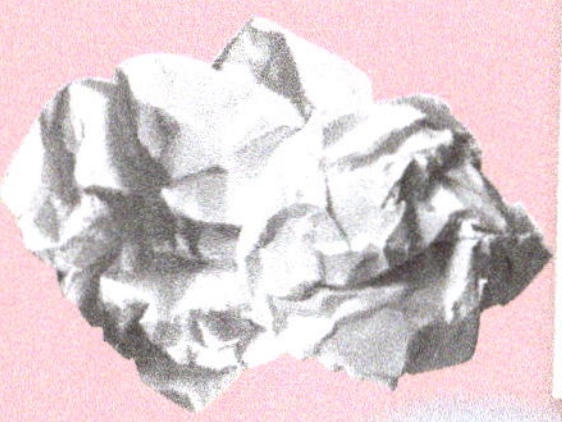

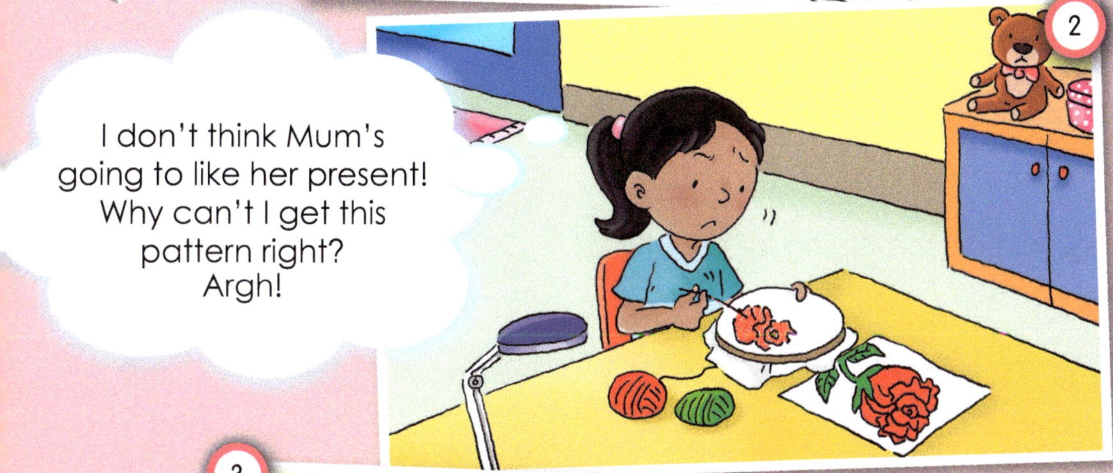

2. *I don't think Mum's going to like her present! Why can't I get this pattern right? Argh!*

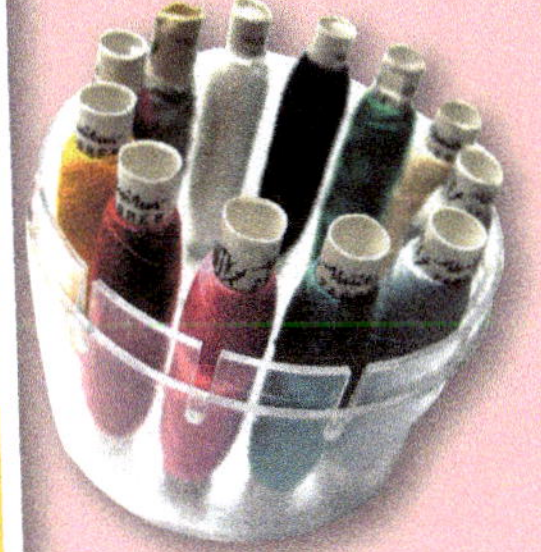

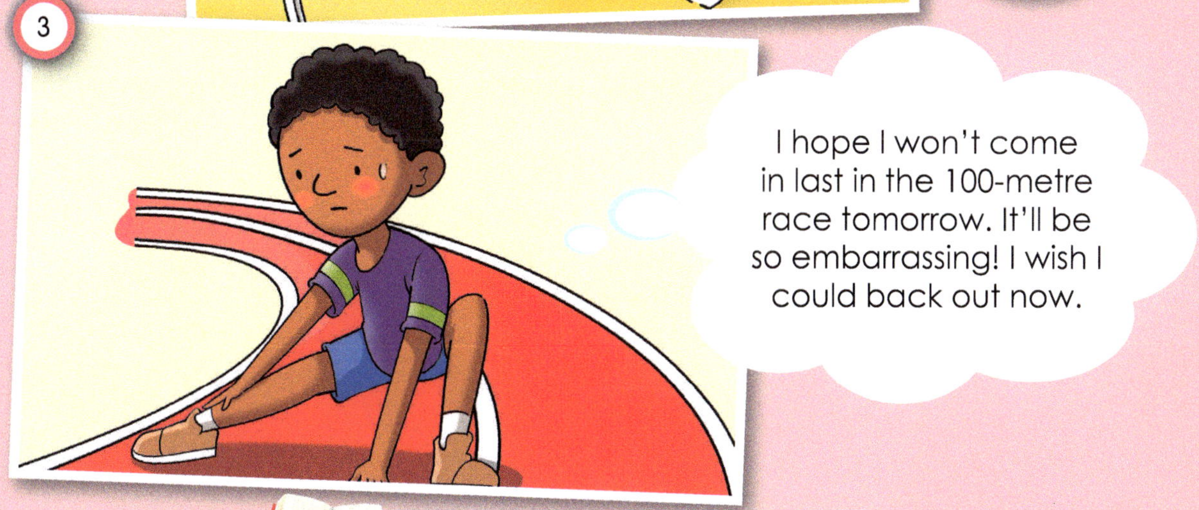

3. *I hope I won't come in last in the 100-metre race tomorrow. It'll be so embarrassing! I wish I could back out now.*

confidence: a strong belief in one's abilities.

Learning Objective: Pupils will be able to understand how different emotions can affect them, and recognise and accept individual differences and similarities for a positive self-esteem.

51

 Haris, Tawan and Ajit do not feel confident about themselves. They are filled with negative thoughts. Examine the following thoughts and put a tick in the boxes of those that will make them more confident.

No one can help me. ☐

My classmates will laugh at my ideas. ☐

I can see if Lam can help me with my presentation since he's so good at these things! ☐

I should just practise more. The better I know the information, the more confident I'll be. ☐

The class will be bored listening to me. ☐

I can ask Eileen for help. ☐

Mother will be disappointed by how untidy this looks. ☐

I'm useless. I can't even do a simple cross-stitch! ☐

I can watch how they do this on the Internet. ☐

Mother will be able to see I've tried my best. She loves it whenever I do something for her anyway! ☐

I've practised hard enough. I should just do my best tomorrow. ☐

Everyone will be looking at me when I come in last in the race. ☐

I may fall tomorrow. It will be so embarrassing! ☐

I should get enough rest tonight so that I can run well tomorrow. ☐

I need to be positive and run to win! ☐

Think positively about yourself. When you are not confident, talk to your family, teachers, school counsellors or your close friends. They can help you with advice and encouragement. Learn to talk positively to yourself too! Be your best supporter!

encouragement: giving emotional support to someone.

Name: Class: Date:

Lesson 2

Our Strengths And Weaknesses

 Decide if each picture shows a superfriend's strength or weakness by drawing either a 🙂 or 🙁 in the circles provided.

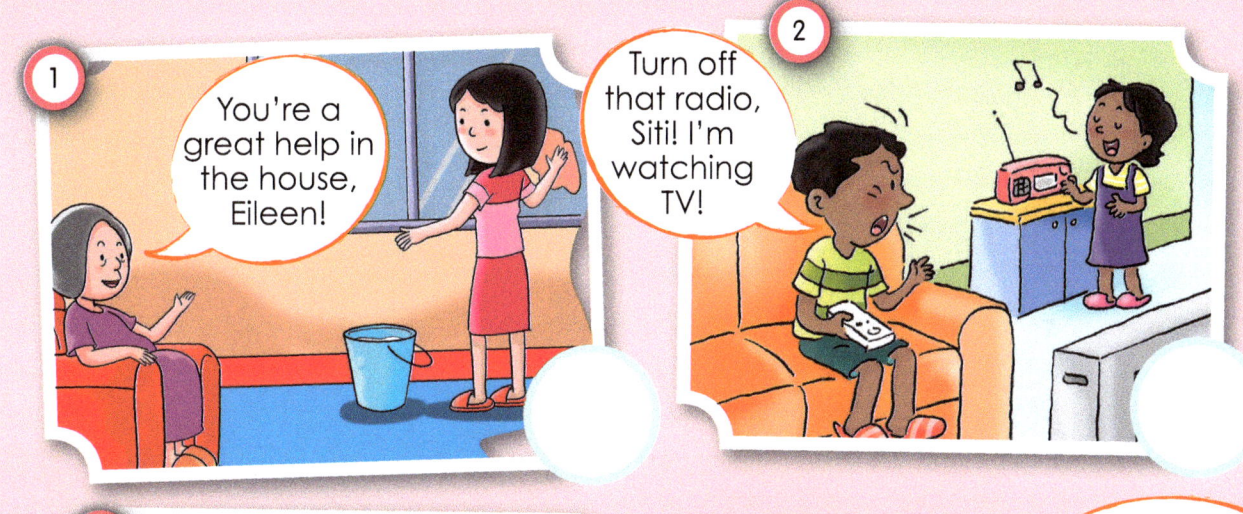

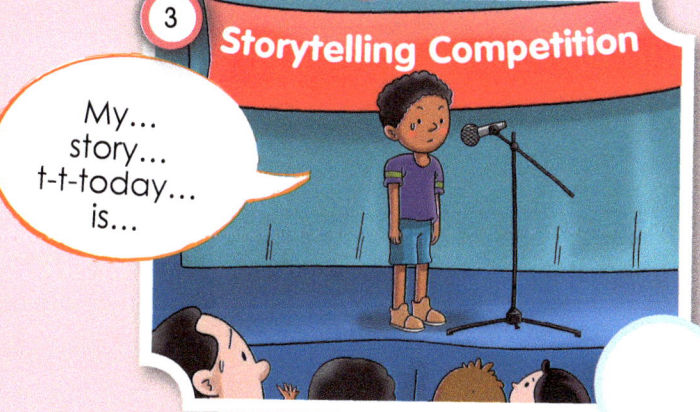

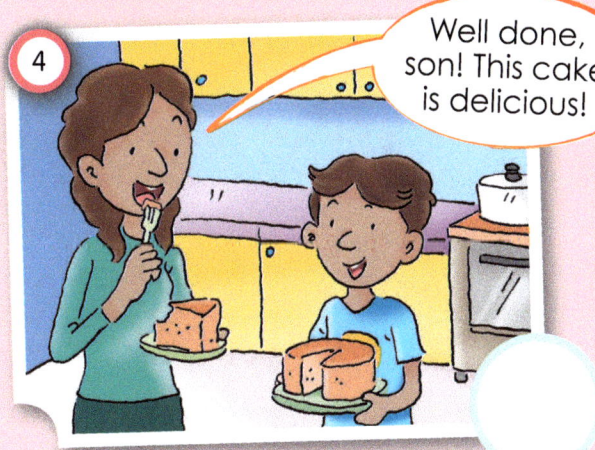

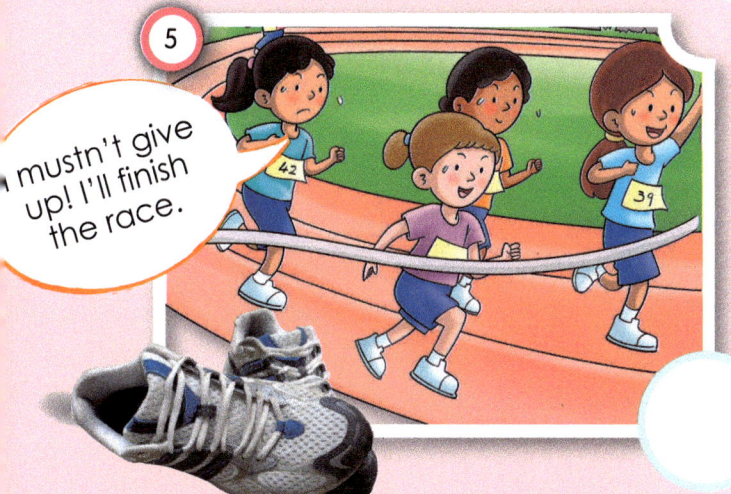

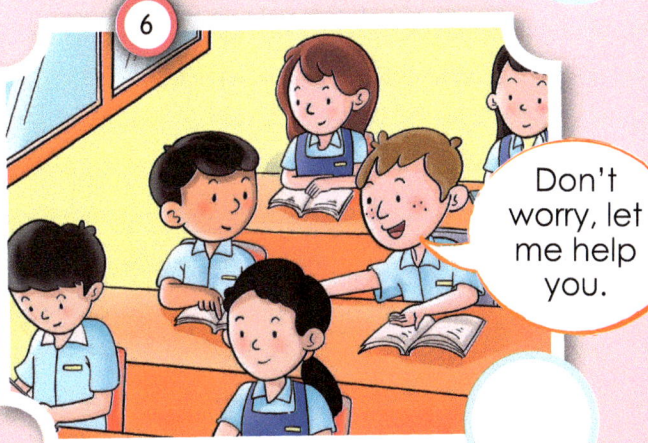

Learning Objective: Pupils will be able to recognise and accept individual differences and similarities for a positive self-esteem, and identify positive ways of managing their emotions.

53

Each of us has our strengths and weaknesses. Knowing what our strengths are will help us be thankful and get better at what we are strong in. When we know our weaknesses, we can learn to overcome or live with them without feeling negative.

> Seek help from family members, teachers, school counsellors and friends!

Describe three of your strengths and say how you can use them to help others.

My strengths

1. _____
2. _____
3. _____

Describe three of your weaknesses and say how you can overcome them.

My weaknesses

1. _____
2. _____
3. _____

Be patient. Overcoming weaknesses takes time and effort. Keep working at it!

Name: Class: Date:

Lesson 3

Try Something New

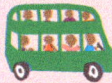 Trying out new things can help build your confidence. What new things are the superfriends doing?

1. 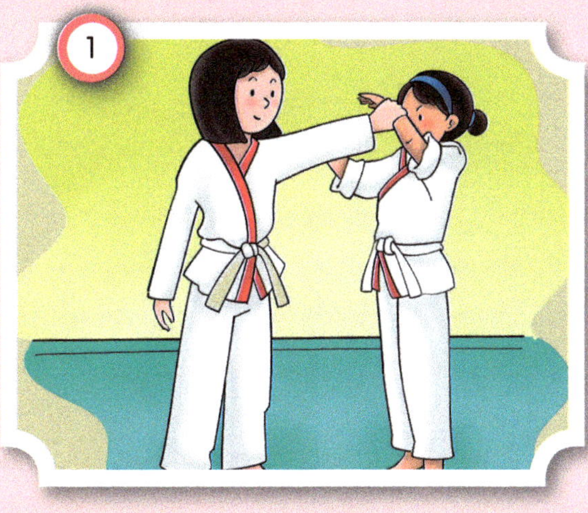
2. 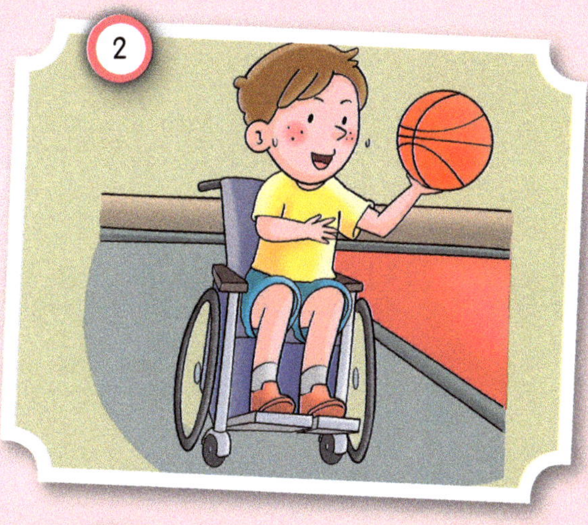
3. 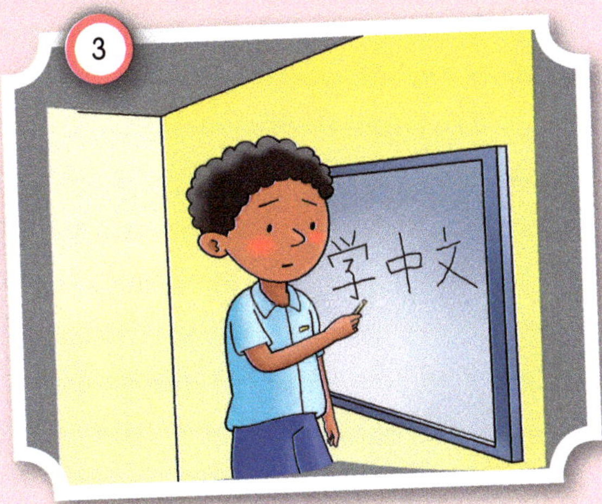
4. 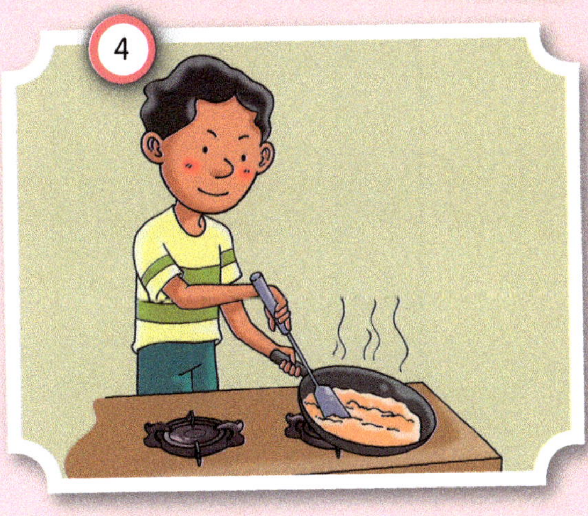
5. 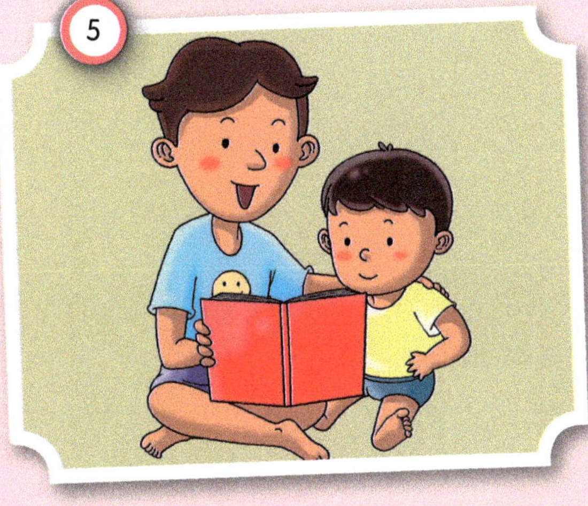
6.

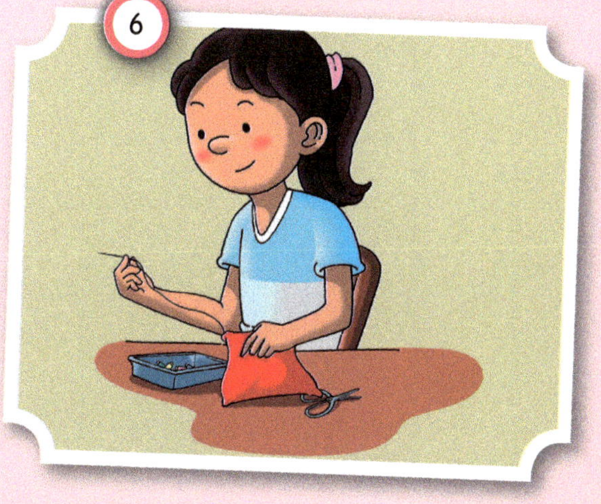

Learning Objective: Pupils will be able to recognise and accept individual differences and similarities for a positive self-esteem, and identify positive ways of managing their emotions.

1. Think of something you are interested in but have never tried. Write about it in the yellow My Goal box at the bottom of the page.
2. Write down two Sub-Goals (blue boxes) that will lead you to your main goal.
3. Describe the challenges (problems) you may face in the orange boxes.
4. Think of the solutions to overcome challenges and write them in the green boxes.

I have reached my goal!

I can overcome it by
_____
_____
_____

I can overcome it by
_____
_____
_____

One challenge I may face is
_____
_____

One challenge I may face is
_____
_____

My sub-goal
_____
_____

My sub-goal
_____
_____

My goal

I want to _____
_____
_____

56

goal: a target that you set, then work to achieve.

Name: **Class:** **Date:** Lesson 4

Caution, Danger Ahead!

 It is important that you learn to protect yourself from dangerous situations. Look at the pictures below and say why there might be danger. Fill in the blanks and read out the advice for each situation.

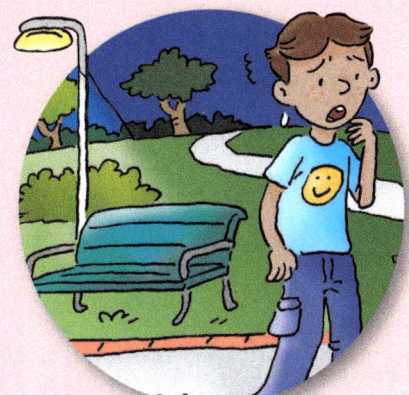

1. Av____ l____ly places.

2. Do not go out a_____ late at n_____.

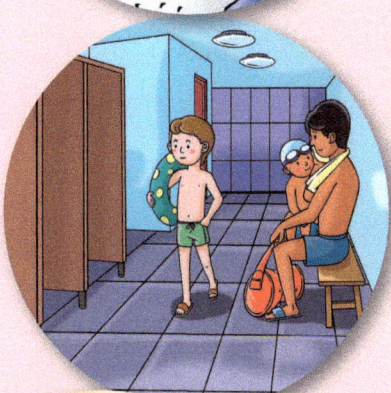

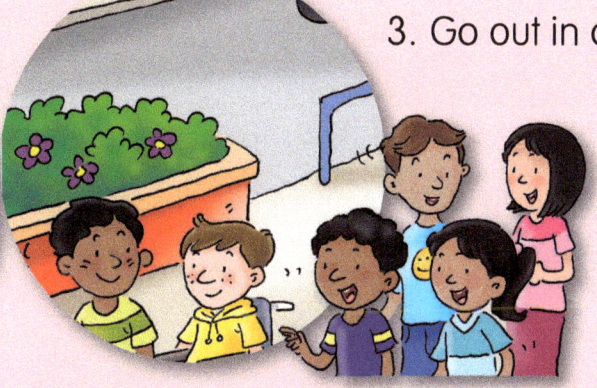

3. Go out in a g_____.

4. Avoid talking to str_____ in the changing rooms of swimming pools.

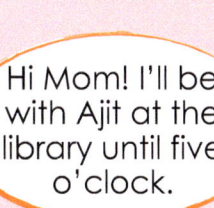

5. Always let your p_____ know w_____ you are going to be.

"Hi Mom! I'll be with Ajit at the library until five o'clock."

Learning Objective: Pupils will be able to seek appropriate sources of help or skills needed when threatened by dangerous situations such as sexual abuse.

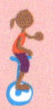 Read the questions below and write your responses in the spaces provided.

1. How do you usually come to school and go home from school?
   _____

2. Who do you usually come to school or go home from school with?
   _____

3. List down two dangerous situations you could possibly encounter on your way to school or on your way home.

   i. _____

   ii. _____

4. If you encounter danger while on the public bus, who would you approach for help and why?
   _____
   _____
   _____

5. Name the adult(s) you usually go out with. What is their relationship to you?

   Name: _____ Relationship: _____

   Name: _____ Relationship: _____

6. List two precautions you can take if you go out without an adult accompanying you.

   i. _____

   ii. _____

Name: Class: Date:

Lesson 5

Protect Yourself

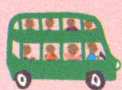 Look at the pictures below.

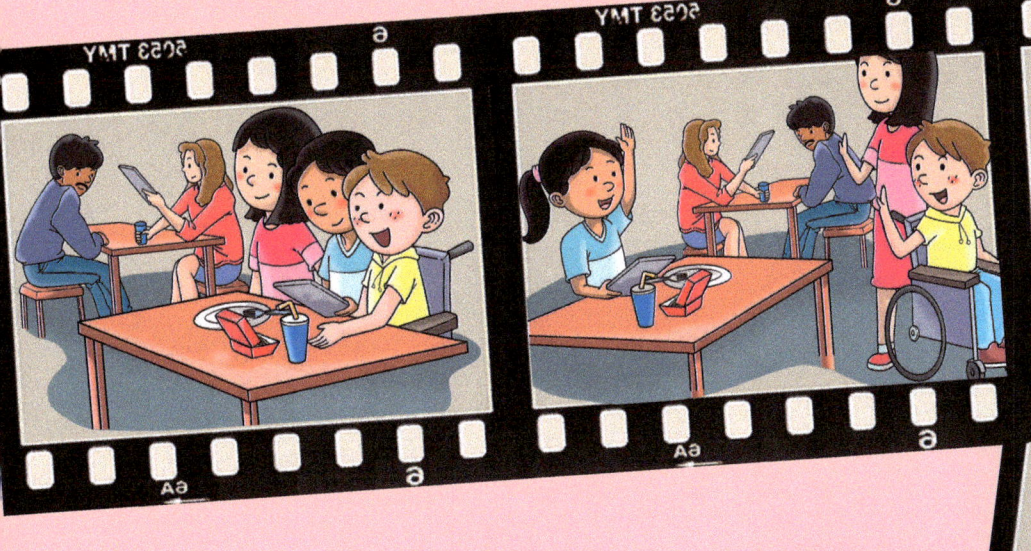

"Young girl, we've just bought a new tablet for our son. Can you help us?"

What do you think Tawan should do? Write your response in the space below.

_____
_____
_____
_____

Learning Objective: Pupils will be able to differentiate between acceptable and unacceptable touch, and seek appropriate sources of help or skills needed when threatened by dangerous situations such as sexual abuse.

59

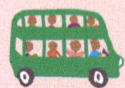

Look at the pictures below. What should Ajit say to Haris? Fill in the speech bubble.

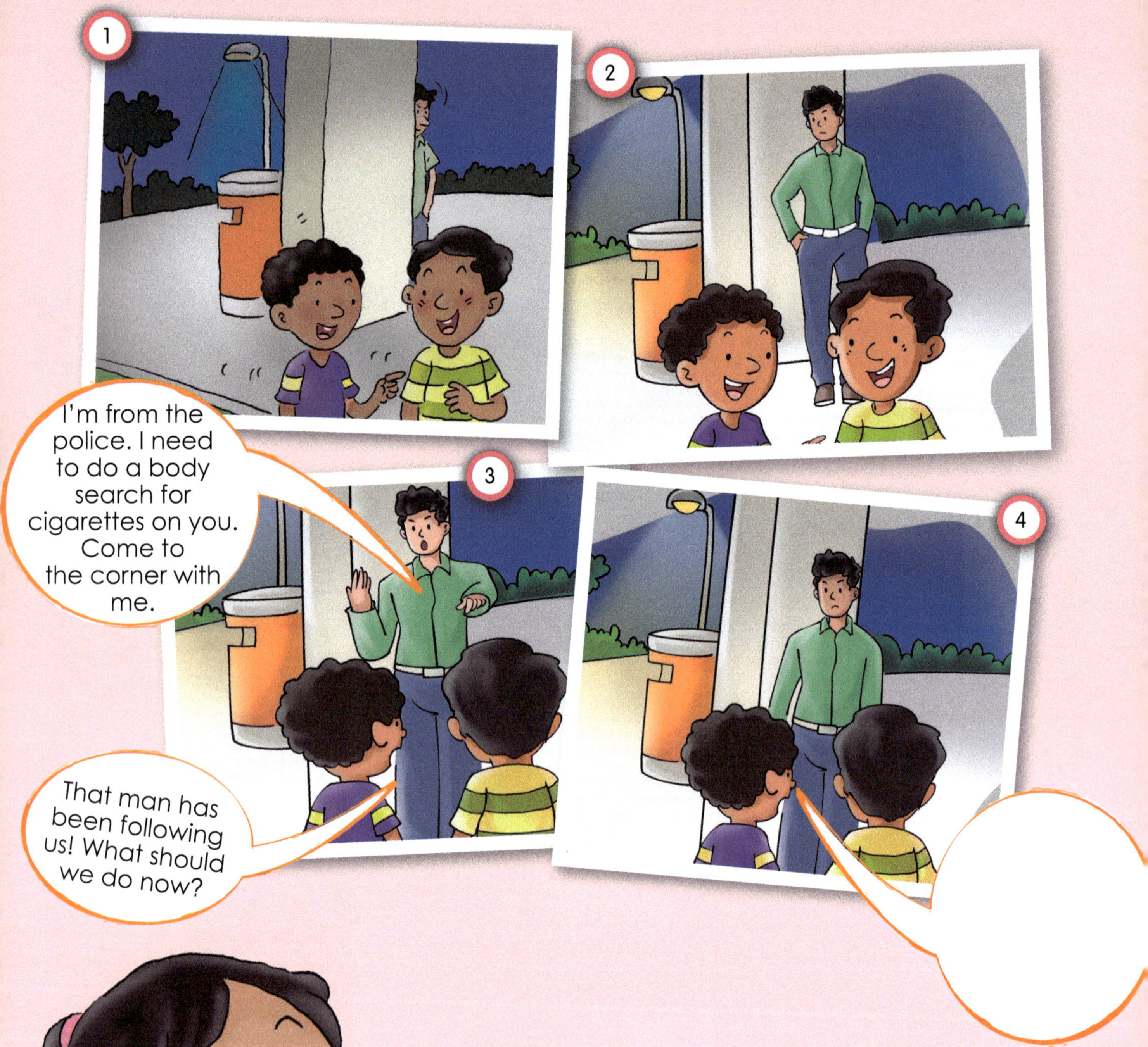

1.

2.

3. "I'm from the police. I need to do a body search for cigarettes on you. Come to the corner with me."

"That man has been following us! What should we do now?"

4.

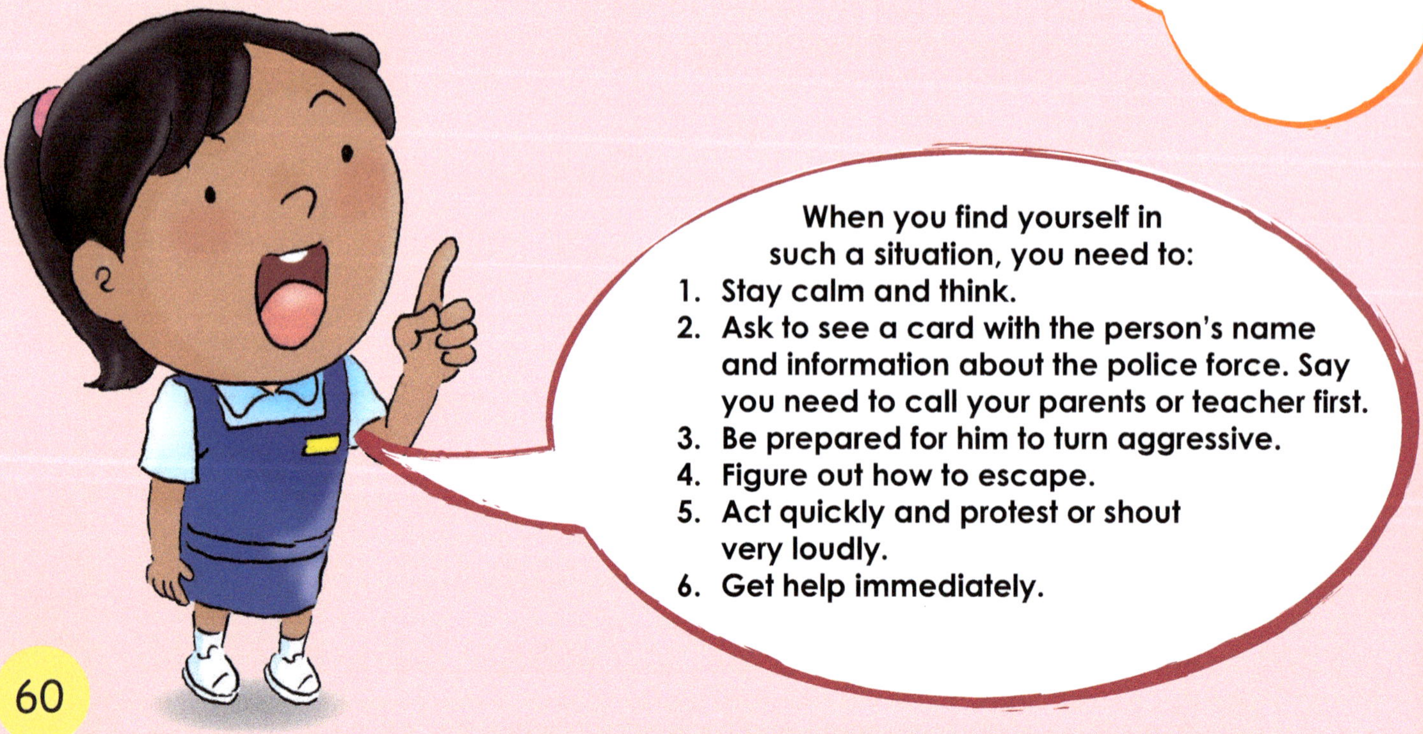

When you find yourself in such a situation, you need to:
1. Stay calm and think.
2. Ask to see a card with the person's name and information about the police force. Say you need to call your parents or teacher first.
3. Be prepared for him to turn aggressive.
4. Figure out how to escape.
5. Act quickly and protest or shout very loudly.
6. Get help immediately.

60

Beware Of Offers From Strangers

Lesson 6

Name: _____ Class: _____ Date: _____

Study the pictures below and discuss the questions with your partner. Then, write your responses in the spaces provided.

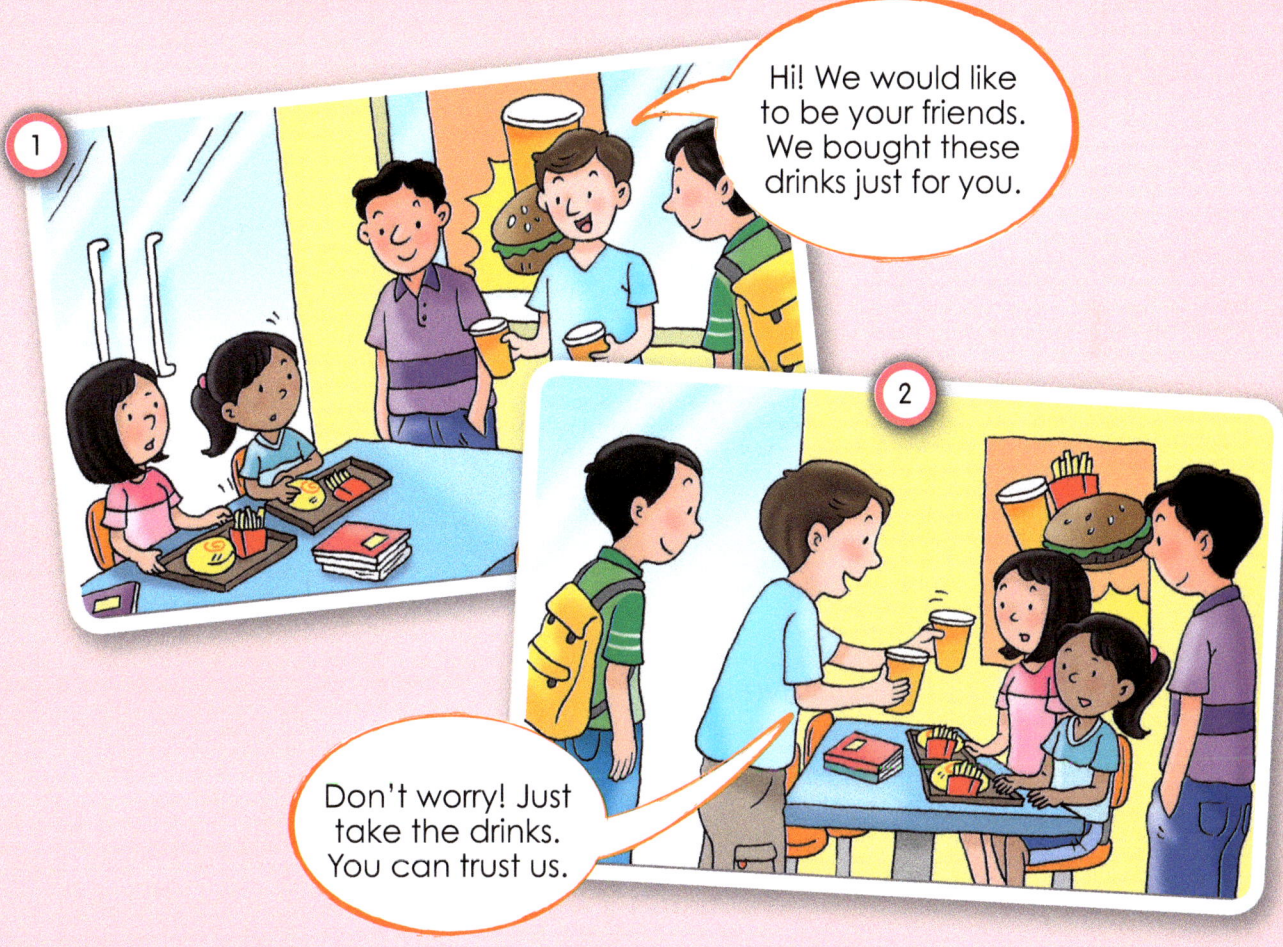

1. Should Tawan and Eileen accept the boys' offer?

   _____

2. What are the dangers of accepting the boys' offer?

   _____
   _____
   _____

Learning Objective: Pupils will be able to seek appropriate sources of help or skills needed when threatened by dangerous situations such as sexual abuse.

3. The three boys will not stop asking Tawan and Eileen to accept the drinks they have bought. What do you think Tawan and Eileen can do?

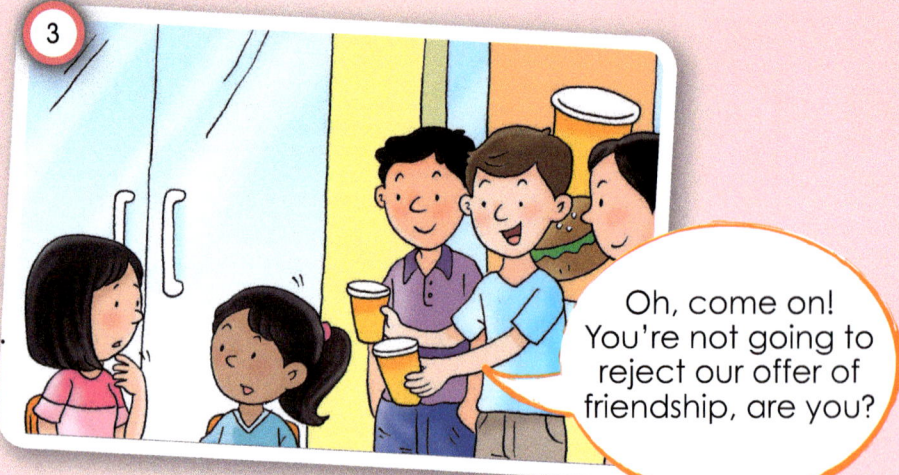

Oh, come on! You're not going to reject our offer of friendship, are you?

_____

_____

_____

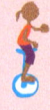 You can learn to be responsible for your own safety by staying alert to the dangers of sexual abuse around you.

Write down what you have learnt from this lesson.

_____

_____

_____

_____

List down two places where you need to take extra care of your food and drinks.

1. _____ 2. _____

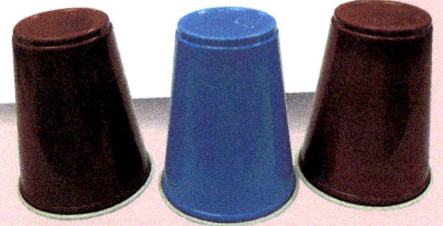

Name: Class: Date: Lesson 7

What Should I Do?

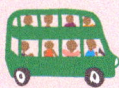 Haris was very uncomfortable about something that happened to him this afternoon. He felt he had to tell somebody, so he texted Harold in the evening.

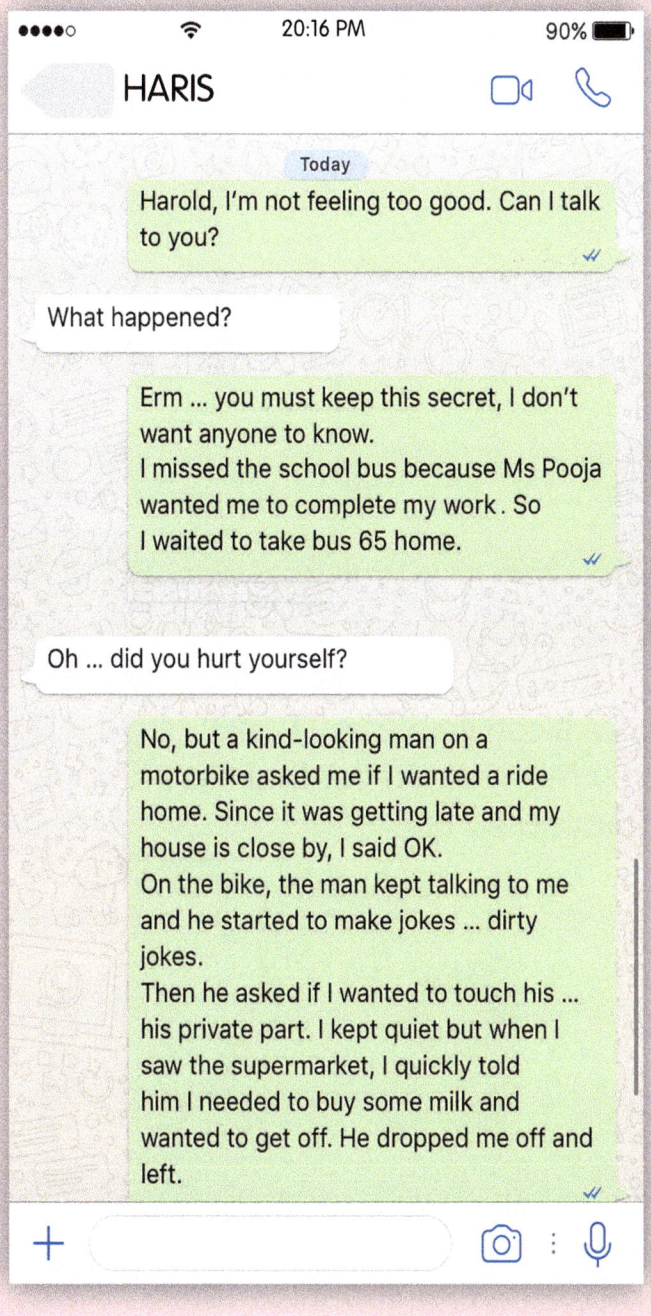

HARIS

Today

Harold, I'm not feeling too good. Can I talk to you?

What happened?

Erm ... you must keep this secret, I don't want anyone to know.
I missed the school bus because Ms Pooja wanted me to complete my work. So I waited to take bus 65 home.

Oh ... did you hurt yourself?

No, but a kind-looking man on a motorbike asked me if I wanted a ride home. Since it was getting late and my house is close by, I said OK.
On the bike, the man kept talking to me and he started to make jokes ... dirty jokes.
Then he asked if I wanted to touch his ... his private part. I kept quiet but when I saw the supermarket, I quickly told him I needed to buy some milk and wanted to get off. He dropped me off and left.

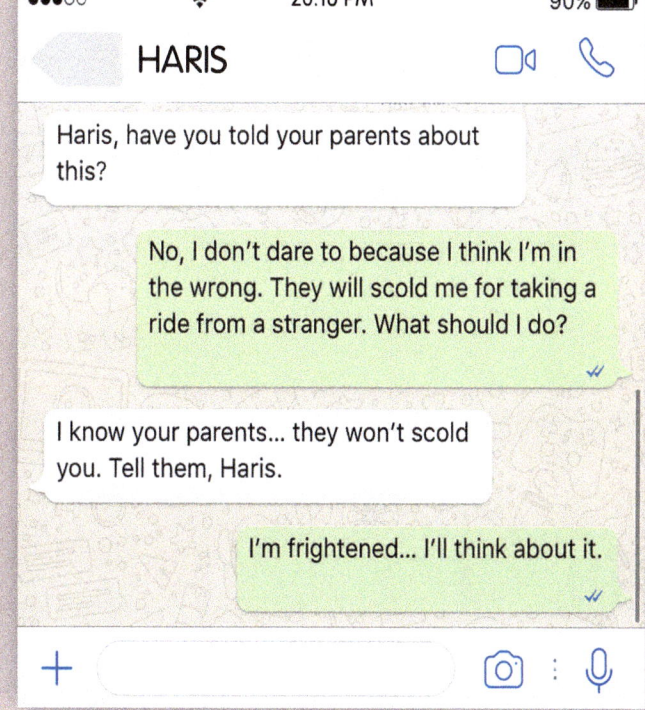

HARIS

Haris, have you told your parents about this?

No, I don't dare to because I think I'm in the wrong. They will scold me for taking a ride from a stranger. What should I do?

I know your parents... they won't scold you. Tell them, Haris.

I'm frightened... I'll think about it.

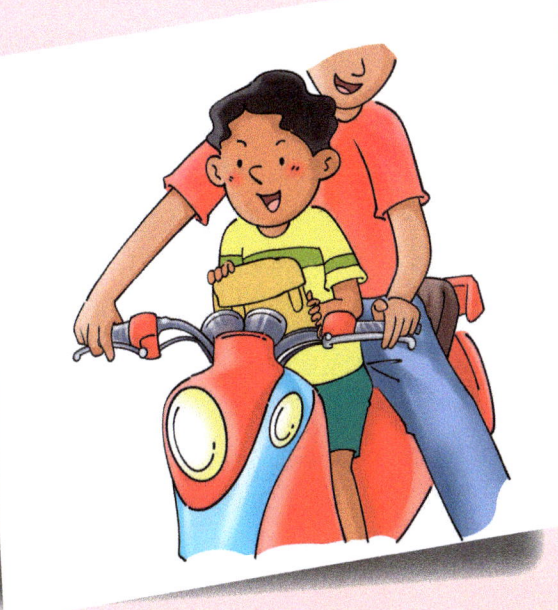

Learning Objective: Pupils will be able to seek appropriate sources of help or skills needed when threatened by dangerous situations such as sexual abuse.

63

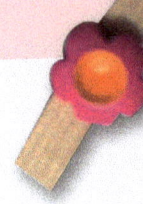

Discuss the following questions with your partner and write your answers in the spaces provided.

1. Should Haris tell his parents what happened? Why or why not?

   _____
   _____
   _____

2. Should Haris blame himself?

   _____
   _____
   _____

3. What can Haris do if he sees the man who gave him a ride again?

   _____
   _____

Sexual abuse can happen to anyone—both boys and girls. It can come from a stranger or someone you know. It can cause you to feel afraid, embarrassed and guilty. However, you must remember that it is not your fault. No one should touch you inappropriately or make you feel uncomfortable.

If you have been sexually abused, talk to an adult whom you trust. Tell them what happened.

Sexual abuse is a criminal offence and the offender must be punished. Go with an adult (your parents, teacher or someone you trust) to make a police report. Many people are ready to help and support you.

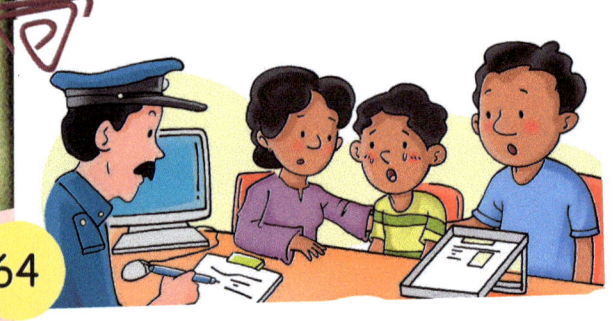

64

NEW WORDS

Lesson: Date:

MY LESSON TODAY ...
(Write down the things you remember.)

Lesson: Date:

MY LESSON TODAY ...
(Write down the things you remember.)

Lesson: Date:

MY LESSON TODAY ...
(Write down the things you remember.)

Lesson: Date:

MY LESSON TODAY ...
(Write down the things you remember.)

Lesson: Date:

MY LESSON TODAY ...
(Write down the things you remember.)

MY LEARNING LOG

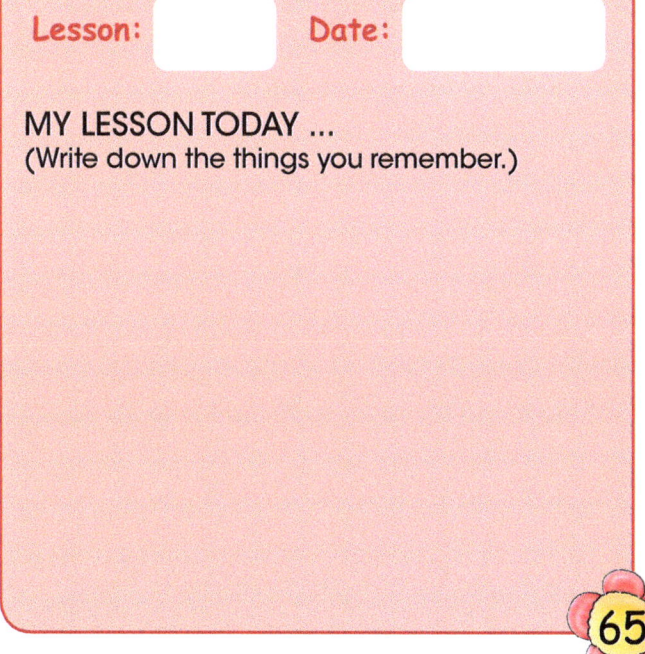

MY LEARNING LOG

NEW WORDS

Lesson: _____ Date: _____

MY LESSON TODAY …
(Write down the things you remember.)

Lesson: _____ Date: _____

MY LESSON TODAY …
(Write down the things you remember.)

Lesson: _____ Date: _____

MY LESSON TODAY …
(Write down the things you remember.)

Lesson: _____ Date: _____

MY LESSON TODAY …
(Write down the things you remember.)

Lesson: _____ Date: _____

MY LESSON TODAY …
(Write down the things you remember.)

NEW WORDS

Lesson: **Date:**

MY LESSON TODAY ...
(Write down the things you remember.)

Lesson: **Date:**

MY LESSON TODAY ...
(Write down the things you remember.)

Lesson: **Date:**

MY LESSON TODAY ...
(Write down the things you remember.)

Lesson: **Date:**

MY LESSON TODAY ...
(Write down the things you remember.)

Lesson: **Date:**

MY LESSON TODAY ...
(Write down the things you remember.)

MY LEARNING LOG

MY LEARNING LOG

NEW WORDS

Lesson: Date:

MY LESSON TODAY ...
(Write down the things you remember.)

Lesson: Date:

MY LESSON TODAY ...
(Write down the things you remember.)

Lesson: Date:

MY LESSON TODAY ...
(Write down the things you remember.)

Lesson: Date:

MY LESSON TODAY ...
(Write down the things you remember.)

Lesson: Date:

MY LESSON TODAY ...
(Write down the things you remember.)

NEW WORDS

Lesson: ____ Date: ____

MY LESSON TODAY ...
(Write down the things you remember.)

Lesson: ____ Date: ____

MY LESSON TODAY ...
(Write down the things you remember.)

Lesson: ____ Date: ____

MY LESSON TODAY ...
(Write down the things you remember.)

Lesson: ____ Date: ____

MY LESSON TODAY ...
(Write down the things you remember.)

Lesson: ____ Date: ____

MY LESSON TODAY ...
(Write down the things you remember.)

MY LEARNING LOG

MY LEARNING LOG

NEW WORDS

Lesson: Date:

MY LESSON TODAY ...
(Write down the things you remember.)

Lesson: Date:

MY LESSON TODAY ...
(Write down the things you remember.)

Lesson: Date:

MY LESSON TODAY ...
(Write down the things you remember.)

Lesson: Date:

MY LESSON TODAY ...
(Write down the things you remember.)

Lesson: Date:

MY LESSON TODAY ...
(Write down the things you remember.)